Practical
Forensic
Medicine and
Toxicology

Practical
Forensic
Medicine and
Toxicology

KK Banerjee MBBS, MD
Professor
Department of Forensic Medicine and Toxicology
University College of Medical Sciences and
Guru Tegh Bahadur Hospital, Delhi

Professor and Head
Department of Forensic Medicine and Toxicology
Faculty of Medical Sciences
University of Delhi, Delhi

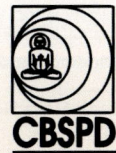

CBSPD

CBS Publishers & Distributors Pvt Ltd

New Delhi • Bengaluru • Chennai • Kochi • Kolkata • Lucknow • Mumbai
Hyderabad • Jharkhand • Nagpur • Patna • Pune • Uttarakhand

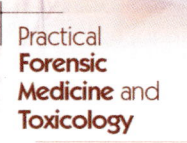

Practical
Forensic
Medicine and
Toxicology

ISBN: 978-93-88178-84-6

Copyright © Author and Publisher

First Edition: 2019
   Reprint: 2024

All rights reserved. No part of this book may be reproduced or transmitted in any form or by any means, electronic or mechanical, including photocopying, recording, or any information storage and retrieval system without permission, in writing, from the author and the publisher.

Published by Satish Kumar Jain and produced by Varun Jain for

CBS Publishers & Distributors Pvt Ltd
4819/XI Prahlad Street, 24 Ansari Road, Daryaganj, New Delhi 110 002
Ph: 011-23289259, 23266861   Website: www.cbspd.com
                                              e-mail: delhi@cbspd.com

Corporate Office: 204 FIE, Industrial Area, Patparganj, Delhi 110 092
Ph: 011-4934 4934   Fax: 011-4934 4935   e-mail: publishing@cbspd.com; publicity@cbspd.com

Branches

• **Bengaluru:** Seema House 2975, 17th Cross, KR Road, Banasankari 2nd Stage, Bengaluru 560 070, Karnataka, India
  Ph: +91-80-26771678/79   Fax: +91-80-26771680   e-mail: bangalore@cbspd.com
• **Chennai:** 7, Subbaraya Street, Shenoy Nagar, Chennai 600 030, Tamil Nadu, India
  Ph: +91-44-26680620, 26681266   Fax: +91-44-42032115   e-mail: chennai@cbspd.com
• **Kochi:** 42/1325, 1326, Power House Road, Opp KSEB, Power House, Ernakulum Kochi 682 018, Kerala, India
  Ph: +91-484-4059061-65,67   Fax: +91-484-4059065   e-mail: kochi@cbspd.com
• **Kolkata:** 147, Hind Ceramics Compound, 1st Floor, Nilgunj Road, Belghoria, Kolkata-700056, West Bengal, India
  Ph: +91-9096713055/7798394118, 9836841399   e-mail: kolkata@cbspd.com
• **Lucknow:** Basement, Khushnuma Complex, 7 Meerabai Marg (Behind Jawahar Bhawan),Lucknow-226001, UP, India
  Ph: +0522-4000032   e-mail: tiwari.lucknow@cbspd.com
• **Mumbai:** PWD Shed, Gala no 25/26, Ramchandra Bhatt Marg, Next to JJ Hospital Gate no. 2, Opp. Union Bank of India, Noorbaug, Mumbai-400009, Maharashtra, India
  Ph: 022-66661880/89   e-mail: mumbai@cbspd.com

Representatives

• Hyderabad	0-9885175004	• Jharkhand	0-9811541605	• Nagpur	0-8692091830
• Patna	0-9334159340	• Pune	0-9664372571	• Uttarakhand	0-9716462459

Printed at HT Media Ltd, Greater Noida, UP, India

to
my respected and beloved parents
Late Smt Maya Banerjee
Late Sh HP Banerjee

Foreword

Forensic medicine and toxicology is an important subject of medicine as it helps in administration of justice. It has assumed more significance nowadays as crime is increasing at a rapid pace. With the aid of forensic experts the accused can be punished while an innocent can be saved from the gallows. The subject of forensic medicine and toxicology is practical oriented. There are lots of books touching on theoretical aspects but fewer books are available on practical application.

Dr KK Banerjee is having vast practical experience in the subject and his practical knowledge and this endeavor will be of great help to undergraduates, postgraduates and service doctors. It will help in solving day-to-day problems related to medico-legal issues. The book has nicely described duties of doctors in medicolegal cases.

The chapters on injury reporting, age reporting, reporting of victim and accused of sexual offences and reporting of drunken person have been nicely described.

There is a detailed mention of conduction of postmortem, techniques of removal of various organs, technique of examination of genital organs in both sexes. Hardly any book mentions examination of transplanted kidney which is good idea of Dr Banerjee. Every doctor doing autopsy should be aware of NHRC guidelines in custodial deaths, DNA profiling and conduction of autopsies on fetus. There are photographs and diagrams nicely explaining the topics.

Toxicology part also deals concisely but nicely with IPC sections related to poisoning, duties of doctor in poisoning cases, viscera preservation. It also deals with poisons—signs and symptoms, postmortem findings and various medicolegal issues of each poison. Chapters on household poisons and pharmaceutical products are of immense importance.

Dr Banerjee to his wisdom has added chapter on MCI Guidelines for Training in Forensic Medicine and it has been rightly done so. Photographs and diagrams will add to the memory.

I congratulate Prof KK Banerjee for this nice practical edition and wish him success in his endeavor.

DN Bhardwaj
Professor
Forensic Medicine and Toxicology
AIIMS, New Delhi

Preface

The subject of forensic medicine and toxicology is gaining more and more importance after the inclusion of the services of doctors under the purview of Consumer Protection Act 1986. Doctors are very often dragged to the court by patients and their relatives (sometimes on instigation by the lawyers) for alleged medical negligence. Therefore, doctors have started practising defensive medicine to safeguard him/her against any litigation escalating the cost of treatment. Proper practical training is necessary for the medical students at both undergraduate and postgraduate levels on this subject. Most of the cases of alleged medical negligence is due to lack of knowledge of legal medicine or medical jurisprudence by the clinicians. In this book the chapter on *Guidelines for Doctor in Medicolegal case* has been written with a view to make the clinicians aware of the legal aspects of medicine while dealing with patients or dead bodies.

Chapters on *Clinical Forensic Medicine* like injury reporting, age reporting, drunkenness and sexual offences, *Forensic Pathology* like deaths due to different causes and their interpretation, *Forensic Toxicology* dealing with common poisons have well-illustrated colored pictures along with the text for easy understanding that will help the doctor in arriving at a correct final conclusion. The chapter on practical aspects of custodial deaths and NHRC guidelines, DNA profiling and MCI guidelines for training in forensic medicine for MBBS and MD students are special feature of this book.

All the 36 chapters of this book is the compilation of the major branches of forensic medicine and toxicology that I have acquired through my personal experience of 35 years in medicolegal field.

I hope that this book will not only be useful for medical students but also for doctors in other disciplines both in government and private institutes and also lawyers.

KK Banerjee

Contents

Section

I

Forensic Medicine

Introduction

The significance of medical science in human welfare is irrefutable and its impact on social systems is multifarious, affecting a wide spectrum of social elements ranging from population dynamics to economic growth rate. One such crucial role that medical science plays is in the social justice system. Medical investigation of crime and accidents, especially those involving hazard to human welfare or life, is essential in providing invaluable insights on it and occupies a critical position in providing justice to victims or their kin.

The knowledge of practical aspects of the subject of forensic medicine and legal medicine is therefore essential for any doctor. This will help delivery of justice in criminal as well as civil cases involving life and limb of a person. The doctor will also save him/her from alleged negligence leading to litigation during the course of treatment or in the event of death of a patient.

Definitions and Branches of Forensic Medicine

Forensic medicine is a branch of science which deals with the application of medical knowledge for administration of justice.

Medical jurisprudence or legal medicine (Latin Juris: Law, Prudence: Knowledge) is the application of the knowledge of law for the practice of medicine as regulated by a state.

After obtaining a registered degree of MBBS, a doctor gets legal rights, privileges, and obligations to practice medicine as per the defined law of that country. Doctors should therefore update his/her knowledge of the rules and regulations enacted by the state and central government from time to time to avoid injustice because of ignorance of such laws.

From the practical point of view the three main branches of forensic medicine are:
1. Clinical forensic medicine
2. Forensic pathology
3. Forensic toxicology.

Clinical forensic medicine deals with application of medical knowledge for the investigation of cases involving living person.

Examples of such cases are:
a. Injury reporting
b. Age reporting
c. Drunkenness or intoxication
d. Sexual offence
e. Identification
f. Human rights violation
g. Divorce due to medical reasons
h. Insanity

Forensic pathology deals with the postmortem examination of dead bodies to know the pathological process or changes in the person's body leading to death. The causes of death can be
a. Natural death due to aging or illness.
b. Unnatural or suspicious death due to injuries or poisoning which can be suicidal, homicidal (including infanticide) or accidental in nature.

Toxicology is a branch of science which deals with the study of properties, mode of action, fatal dose, signs and symptoms, treatment in living and postmortem findings in case of death of the person because of alleged poisonous substance.

In medical profession every doctor irrespective of the specialty is confronted with a medicolegal case during the course of his/her medical practice regardless of him/her working in government or private hospital/clinic.

A doctor should, therefore, not only have sufficient knowledge of medicine as a general physician or the discipline he/she specializes in but also the legal implications of a particular case. The doctors are often summoned by the court as expert witness to give their evidence in a medicolegal case. In many such cases the verdict of the case solely depends on the opinion of the doctor and punishment to an innocent person can be avoided.

It is for this reason that forensic medicine is one of the important subjects in undergraduate medical curriculum. After the medical profession was brought into the ambit of Consumer Protection Act in 1995, the doctors are forced to practice defensive medicine as they have become vulnerable to litigation by the patients alleging negligence against a doctor.

Unfortunately there is hardly any undergraduate training in the field of forensic medicine in this country. There are many medical institutions in our country where even postgraduates lack practical training as postmortem facilities are not available in their department of forensic medicine.

Medicolegal case (MLC) is one where the doctor after taking history and clinical examination of a case deems it fit to be investigated by the legal authorities for the causation of injury, illness or death of a person.

It is mandatory for the doctor to inform police about a MLC falling under the jurisdiction of the area where the hospital/nursing home/clinic belongs.

Guidelines for Doctors in Medicolegal Case

- In any medicolegal case (MLC) an informed written consent/thumb impression of the patient or relative is required before examining a person, otherwise the doctor may be charged for assault by the person.
- A case brought several days after the actual incident can still be registered as MLC if foul play is suspected.
- Any admitted non-MLC case can be converted into an MLC case if some foul play is suspected by the doctor during the course of treatment.
- In a case of poisoning, the doctor should preserve the vomitus or gastric lavage to avoid charge of causing disappearance of evidence under Section 201 IPC against the treating doctor.
- Any married woman dying as a result of harassment or cruelty by her husband or relative of the husband within seven years of her marriage in relation to dowry demand should be reported by the attending doctor to the police which is dealt under Section 304B IPC (dowry death).
- If death is inevitable in an MLC, arrangement should be made by the doctor to inform the IO (investigation officer)/police/magistrate of the case to record the dying declaration of the person. The attending physician can also record the dying declaration if there is a delay in the arrival of the IO.
- In case of discharge of an MLC case, police should be informed.
- Where the admitted patient leaves against medical advice (LAMA), the police should be informed before discharge.
- Unfortunately if the person does not survive in an MLC, death certificate should not be issued by the treating doctor of a hospital, nursing home or clinic. The dead body should be handed over to the police after taking a receipt and not to the relatives of the deceased. The body is sent by the IO to the mortuary of the hospital for post-mortem examination.
- In case of suicide survivors it is not mandatory for the doctor to report to the police and make it an MLC case; however, it is safe to do so.
- Any registered MBBS doctor is eligible to conduct postmortem examination of a dead body at a center authorized by the competent authority.
- An autopsy surgeon should do a meticulous postmortem examination of a dead body whether or not it is being videographed after receiving the dead body along with complete inquest papers from the IO.
- Postmortem report should be submitted at the earliest to the IO. When the histopathology or viscera has been preserved, the postmortem report can be submitted even without any cause of death. Final cause of death should be given as

and when the histopathology or viscera reports are made available by the IO to the autopsy surgeon.

- All medicolegal reports are confidential documents and therefore should be handed over to the investigating officer (IO) of the case. It cannot be directly handed over to the patient or relatives. However, attested copies of such reports can be given to the relatives if they apply to the concerned authorities of the hospital after paying a requisite fee citing a valid reason, as existing in a particular hospital after obtaining a receipt from the patient or relatives.
- The X-ray films (other than age reporting cases), CT and MRI films are the property of the hospital and cannot be given to the IO of the case unless asked by the court.
- Every clinician should keep a record of the details of history, examination findings, investigation reports, treatment given and day-to-day progress/condition of the patient (if admitted) for his/her own safety and defense in the event of any subsequent litigation, for negligence.
- It is the responsibility of the hospital to keep all medical records up to five years for OPD patients and ten years for indoors in medicolegal cases as per the guidelines laid down by the Director General of Health Services of India.
- Patient's consent is required if any case related to his/her ailment is going to be presented in a conference.
- A doctor is bound to reply in writing under Section 161, CrPC if certain clarification about the case is sought by the IO.
- The police has the authority to summon a doctor in the police station for recording the statement of the doctor during the course of investigation under Section 160, CrPC.
- All MLC cases should be entered in a *Medicolegal Register* for living subjects or *Postmortem Report Form* for dead subjects available in the casualty/forensic medicine department of all Government hospital.
- Every medicolegal report should be written in duplicate. The original should be handed over to the IO of the case after obtaining a receipt and the copy should be maintained in the record of the hospital/nursing home as the case may be. In case of postmortem the original report should be handed over to the IO and copy should be kept in the department of forensic medicine/hospital record department.
- In case of suspected poisoning deaths, a third copy of the postmortem is made which is to be send to the CFSL (central forensic science laboratory) along with the preserved viscera and handed over to the IO of the case.

Injury Reporting

A doctor should be conversant with the following definitions and terms while writing an injury report.

Injury is any harm whatsoever illegally caused to a person's body, mind, reputation and property as defined under Section 44 IPC.

Hurt is any bodily pain, disease or infirmity caused to a person as defined under Section 319 IPC. There is no legal definition of simple injury; however, it is used in place of hurt.

Wound is a breach in the natural continuity of a living tissue.

For practical purposes *injury is classified* as: 1. Simple injury; and 2. Grievous hurt.

Simple injury (not defined by the law) is one which is neither extensive nor severe and heals without leaving a permanent scar.

Examples—contusion and superficial abrasion, superficial incised wound.

Grievous hurt is defined under Section 320 IPC and includes the following eight clauses:

1. Emasculation
2. Permanent privation of sight of either eye
3. Permanent privation of hearing of either ear
4. Privation of any member or joint
5. Destruction or permanent impairment of the powers of any member or joint.
6. Permanent disfiguration of head or face
7. Fracture or dislocation of a bone or tooth.
8. Any hurt:
   a. Which endangers life
   b. Which causes the sufferer to be during the space of twenty days in severe bodily pain.
   c. Unable to follow his/her ordinary pursuits.

Weapon means any thing used, designed to be used or intended for use (a) in causing death or injury to any person, or (b) for the purpose of threatening or intimidating any person, and without restricting the generality of foregoing, includes a firearm. It can be:

1. Sharp-edged weapon
2. Blunt weapon
3. Firearm weapon
4. Any other means such as chemical, burns, poison.

INJURY REPORT PROFORMA

CR No. /A&E No. _____   MLC No._____

Name_____

S/D/W of_____,Age_____Sex_____Religion_____

Residential Address_____Occupation_____

Brought by:

(Name, address of relative or friend)_____

Police Officer: Name_____No. _____

Police Constable: Name_____No. _____

Police Station_____

Date, time and place of examination_____

No. and Date of Police Docket_____	Brief history of the case:
No. and Name of Constable_____	General Physical Examination:
In admitted patient:	Details of Injury/Symptoms
a) Date of admission_____	(in poisoning cases):
b) Date of discharge_____	Injuries:
Articles handed over to police_____	

Injuries table:

Serial No.	Type	Dimensions	Site	Nature	Age	Weapon used	Any other remarks

Consent from the subject:

      Signature/LTI/RTI

Poisoning :   Signs and symptoms.

_____

Identification Marks:

1) _____

2) _____

Details of sample preserved and investigation asked for:

Articles handed over to police_____

Opinion:_____

Signature

Name, Designation and Seal of Doctor

Dangerous weapon is one which is used for cutting, shooting and stabbing. Such as a knife/sharp-edged weapon and firearm weapon. It has been defined as a part of Section 324 IPC.

The following are the various types of injury cases that are reported in a hospital, nursing home, or clinics:

- Road traffic accidents
- Assault by physical violence
- Domestic accidents
- Workplace accidents
- Burn injuries
- Chemical injuries
- Electrical injuries
- Lightning.

Doctors posted in casualty or emergency departments should be efficient both in providing emergency treatment as well as legal formalities for such cases. Centers where such departments are not available, arrangements should be made to shift the patient to higher medical centers at the earliest after giving primary treatment.

EXPLANATION AND INTERPRETATION OF TERMS/POINTS MENTIONED IN THE INJURY REPORT

Consent: An informed consent should be taken in any medicolegal case. The language should be:

"I am willing to undergo medical examination for the various injuries present on my body. I have been explained the nature and consequences of such examination and that the findings may go against my favour."

Identification marks: It should be two in number. Permanent marks preferably on the exposed parts of the body should be noted, such as mole, permanent scar, deformity, tattoos, etc. Exact position should be described with respect to some anatomical landmark on the body.

General physical examination: It includes recording of level of consciousness, pulse, BP, respiratory rate, temperature and other vitals.

Types of injury:
1. Contusion/bruise (Figs 4.1–4.4a and b)
2. Abrasion (Figs 4.5–4.8 and 4.11)
3. Laceration (Fig. 4.12)
4. Stab (Fig. 4.7b)
5. Incised
6. Chop wound
7. Crush injury
8. Avulsion injury
9. Firearm (Figs 4.13a, 4.14b)
10. Dry burn (Figs 4.15a and b)/scald/chemical burns/electrocution or Joule burns (Figs 4.13b and 4.14a).

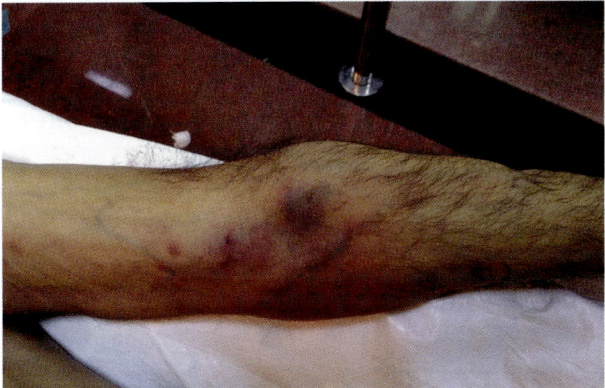

Fig. 4.1: Bruise or contusion

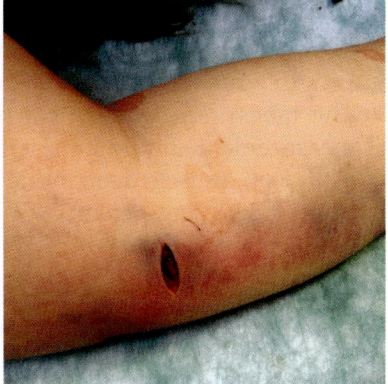

Fig. 4.2: Demonstration of bruise showing staining of subcutaneous tissue

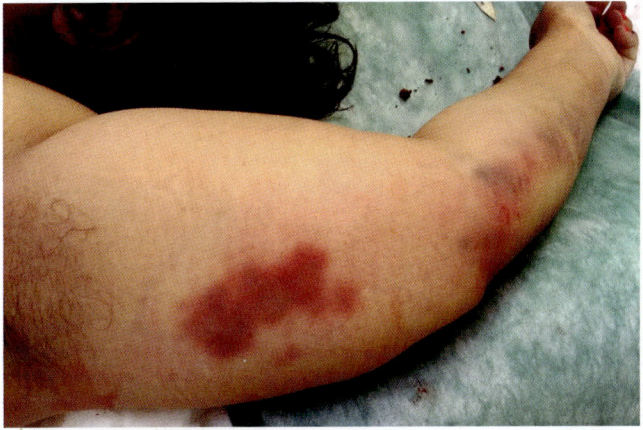

Fig. 4.3: Bruise over upper arm

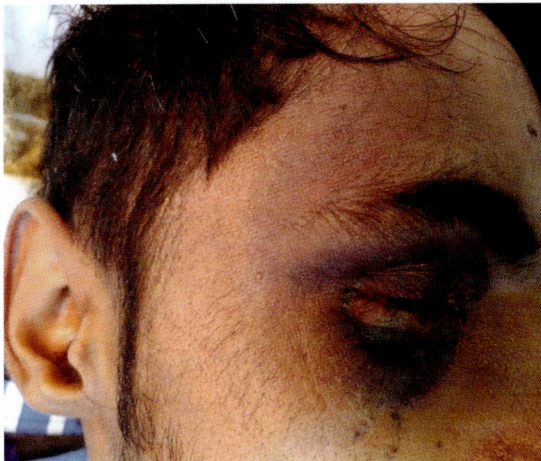

Fig. 4.4a: Black eye—a type of bruise involving the frontal area of the head

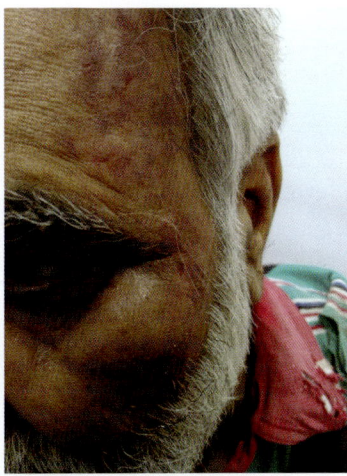

Fig. 4.4b: Hematoma, a kind of bruise, below the outer angle of left eye

Dimensions

- Length × breadth in superficial injuries, such as bruise and abrasion.
- Length × breadth × depth in deep injuries, such as laceration, stab, firearm wounds
  The measurements should be done using a measuring tape or scale. Unit of measurement should be in cm. Depth of an injury should be mentioned as either skin deep, muscle deep, bone deep or cavity and should never be probed into any cavity in a living person as it might create a false tract or injure blood vessel with fatal outcome.

Site/location: Exact location of injury on the body should be with reference to some anatomical landmark such as—abrasion 4 × 5 cm over front of forearm, 3 cm above wrist joint and 6 cm below elbow joint (Figs 4.9 and 4.10).

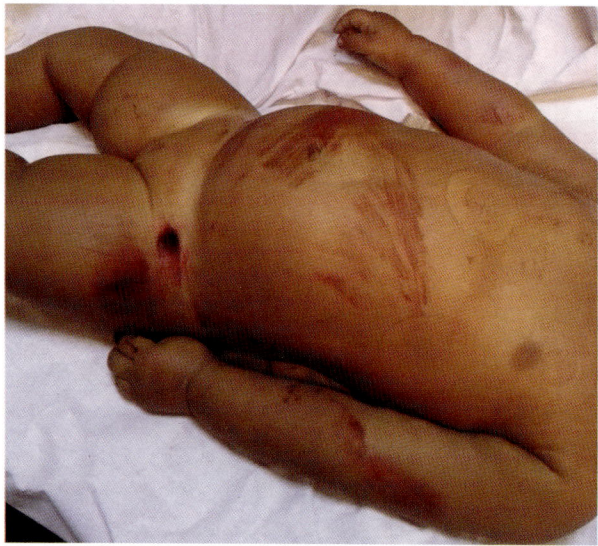

Fig. 4.5: Grazed abrasion

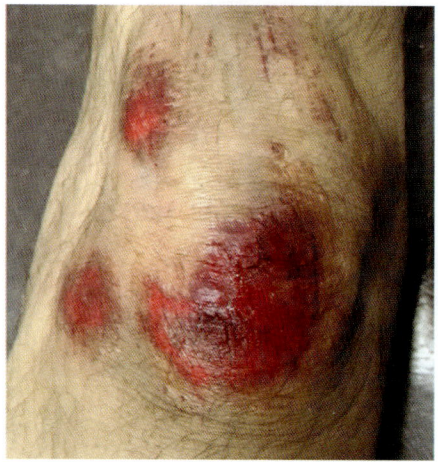

Fig. 4.6a: Fresh abrasion (2 hours old) over knee

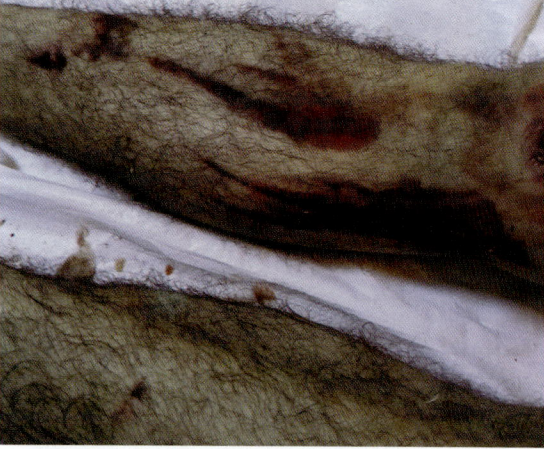

Fig. 4.6b: Abrasion (14 hours old) with dark red adherent scab over right leg below knee

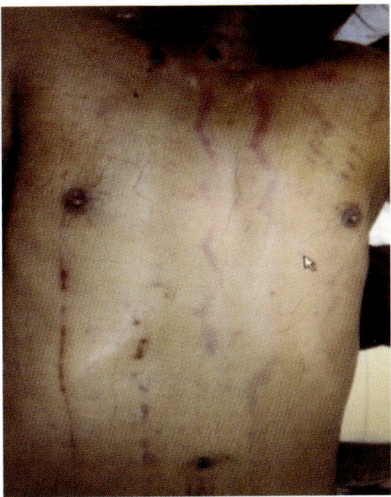

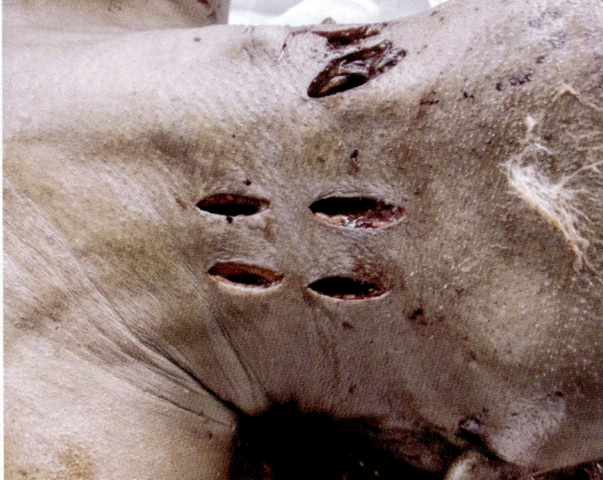

Fig. 4.7a: Tyre mark over front of chest   **Fig. 4.7b:** Multiple stab wounds at the back

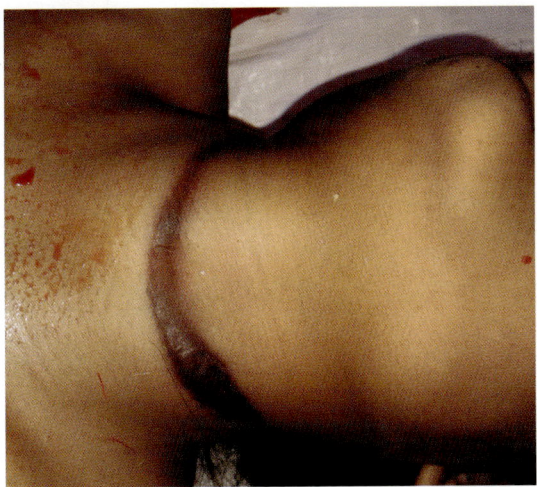

Fig. 4.8: Deep ligature mark (abrasion) around neck in case of hanging

Weapon used: Type of weapon used can be ascertained by close examination of the entry and exit wound (if present) preferably using a magnifying glass in deep injuries and naked eye examination in superficial injuries.

Weapon can be either:
- Sharp edged (single/double edged)
- Blunt weapon
- Firearm weapon.

Age of the injury: Approximate age of the injury depending upon the color changes if it is a bruise and healing process in case of abrasions, laceration, incised wound and burns.

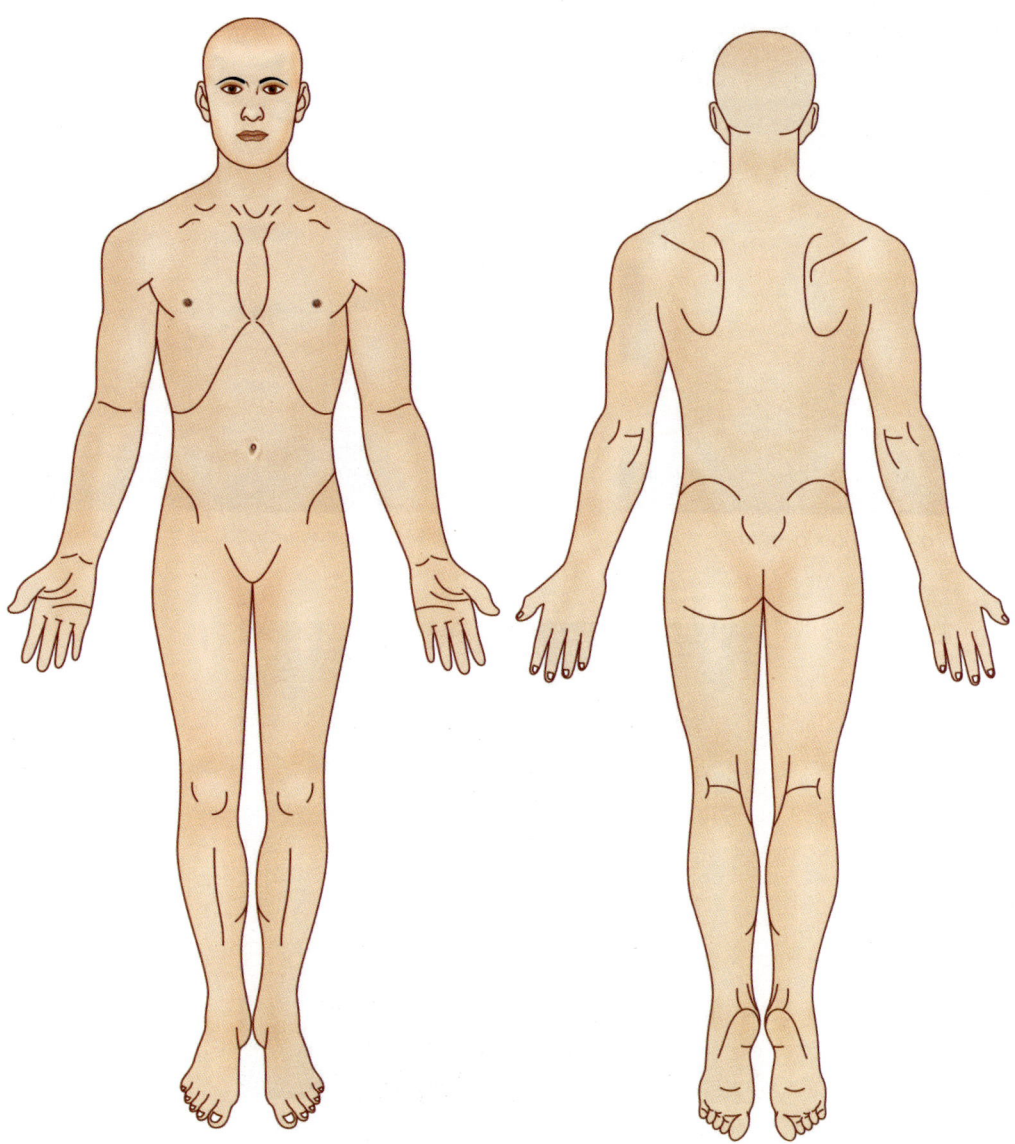

Fig. 4.9: Diagrams to mark various injuries present on the front and back of the body

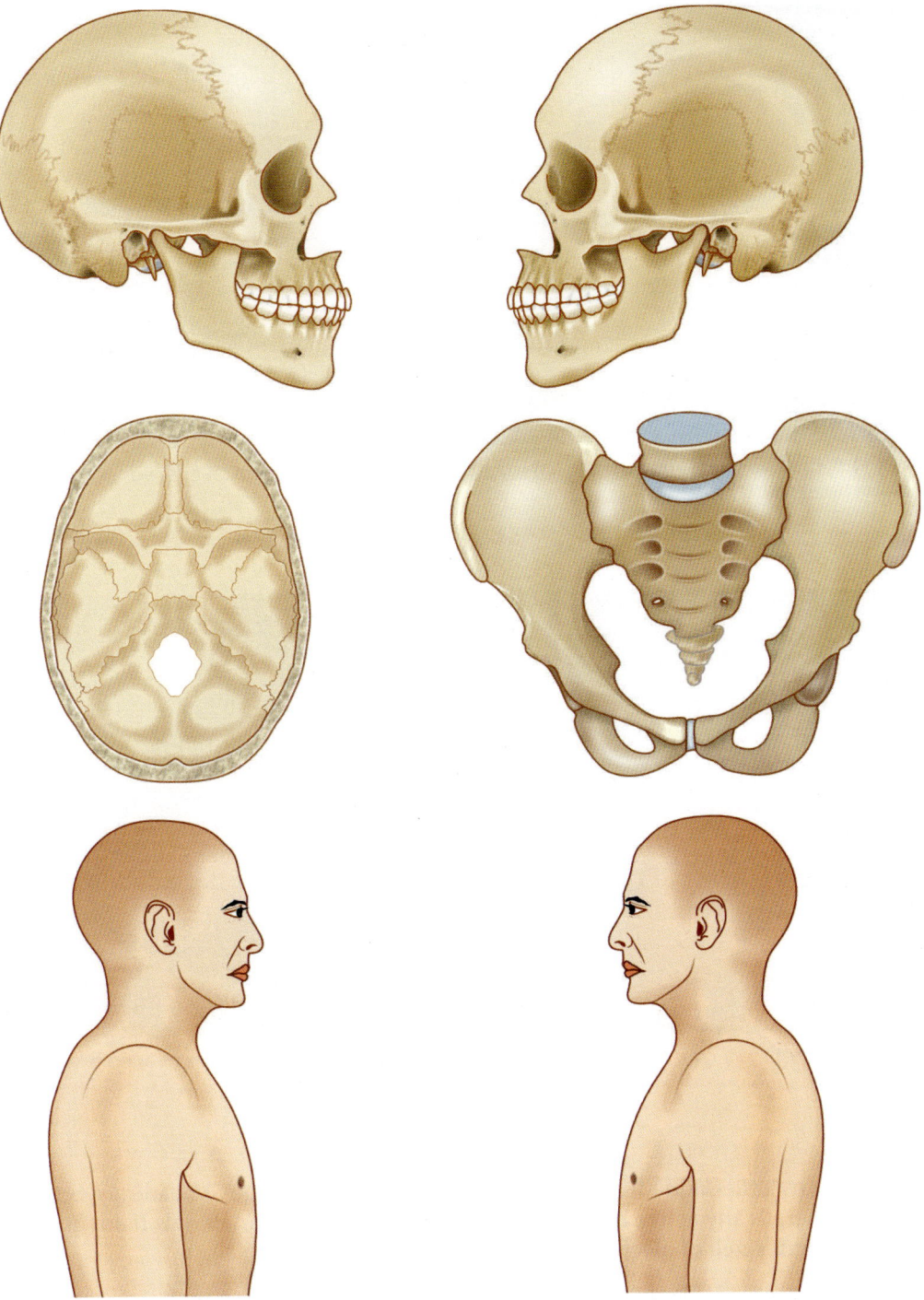

Fig. 4.10: Diagrams to mark various injuries present on skull pelvis and sides of body

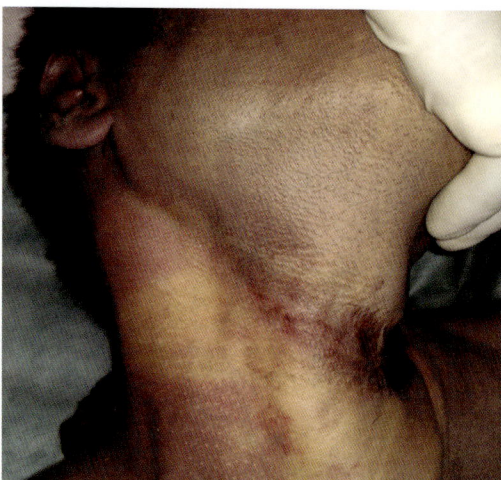

Fig. 4.11: Superficial ligature mark (abrasion) around neck in hanging

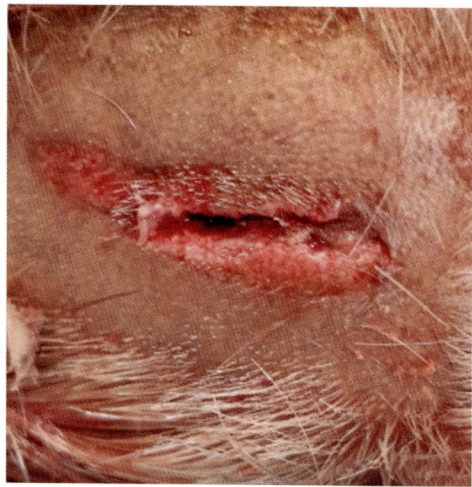

Fig. 4.12: Laceration over vertex of skull

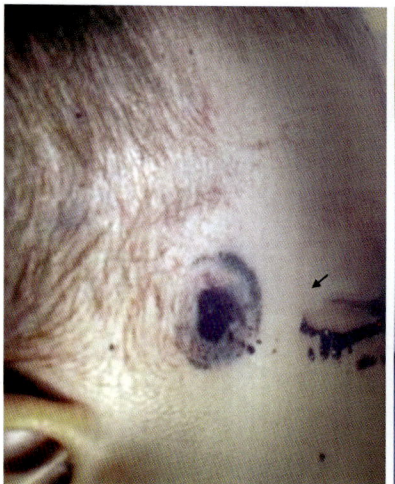

Fig. 4.13a: Bullet injury over temple of skull

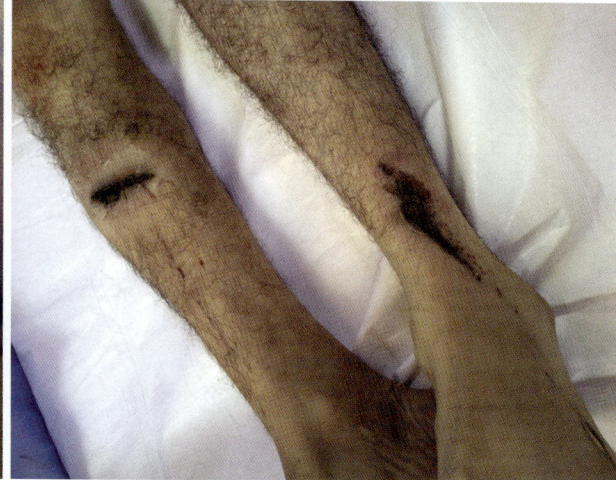

Fig. 4.13b: Electrocution entry mark over both legs

Remarks: Any other added information not included in the above headings. Such as whether there is any active bleeding, stitched wound, foreign materials if any present in the wound, smell of alcohol or any intoxicant.

Samples preserved: Depending upon the case it could be foreign material present on the injured part such as bullet, pellets, broken knife blades.

Investigations asked for: X-ray in cases of suspected fracture of underlying bone, blood and urine for level alcohol or any intoxicant.

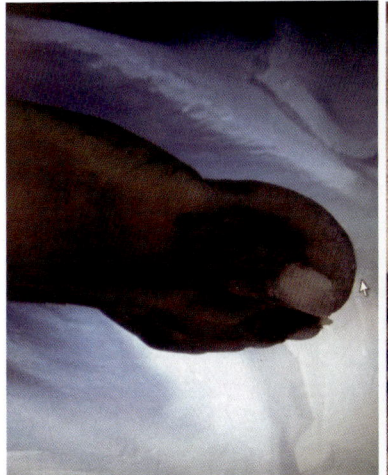

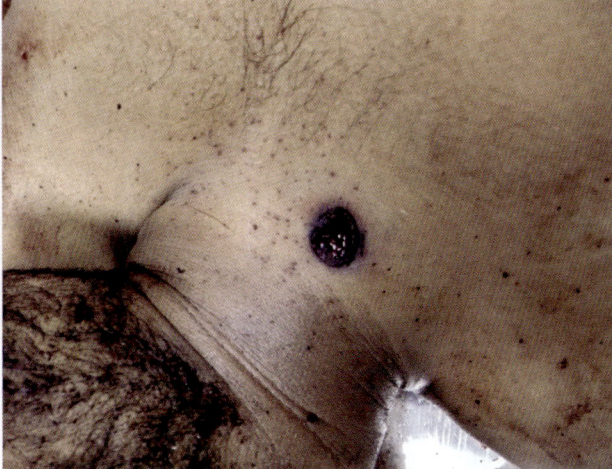

Fig. 4.14a: Electrocution exit point

Fig. 4.14b: Gunshot wounds with tattoing in the surrounding area over back of neck

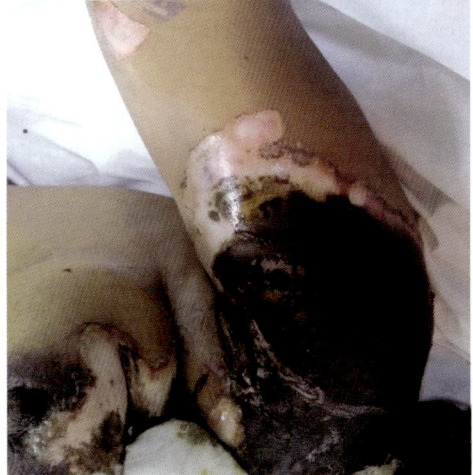

Fig. 4.15a: Antemortem burn showing demarcation between burnt (back) and unburnt (reddish) area

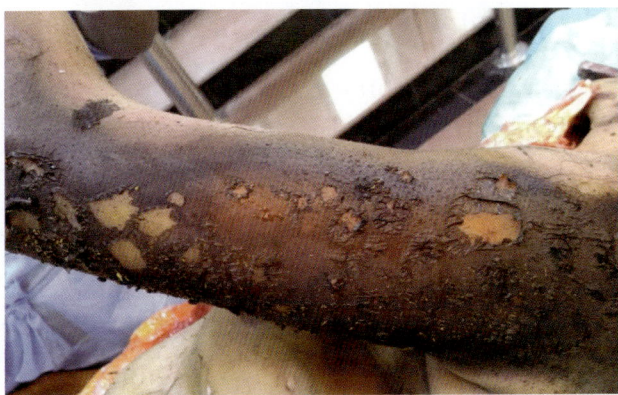

Fig. 4.15b: Postmortem burn. No reddish discoloration under the burnt area of hand

Opinion: "After examining the various injuries present on the body of the subject I am of the opinion that":

- Injury no/s…….. is/are simple in nature caused by a blunt weapon.
- Injury no/s……..is/are grievous in nature caused by a sharp edged/firearm weapon/burns

Depending upon the severity, whether or not the injury/injuries is/are sufficient to cause death in ordinary course of nature should also be mentioned. When investigation report is pending, the opinion should be written as:

Opinion will be given after receiving the report of the investigation when such report is not immediately available. Like in cases of suspected fracture of a bone underlying a bruise.

Subsequent Opinion of Weapon of Offence

Sometimes the alleged weapon of offence is recovered by the police after a few days to a few months after the actual date of a crime and brought to the doctor for opinion. In such cases the alleged weapon should be carefully examined by the doctor and a sketch diagram on a paper should be made mentioning all the dimensions of the alleged weapon. The same should then be compared with the injuries described in the injury report.

Opinion

a. *If it corresponds to injury/injuries present on the body:* The injury/injuries is/are possible with the type of alleged weapon.

b. *If it does not correspond to the injury/injuries present on the body:* The injury/injuries is/are unlikely/not possible with the alleged weapon should be opined. After examination the doctor should sign on the alleged weapon which should be made into a parcel and duly sealed with the seal of the doctor and handed over to the IO after taking a receipt for the same.

The weapon of offence could be:

1. Blunt
   a. Heavy, e.g. big brick or stone, wheels of vehicle, any heavy blunt object (Fig. 4.16)
   b. Light, e.g. thin rod, stick (Fig. 4.17)
2. Sharp
   a. Single edged (Fig. 4.18)
   b. Double edged knife (Fig. 4.18)
   c. Heavy cutting, e.g. axe (Fig. 4.18)
3. Firearm, e.g. shotgun, rifle (Fig. 4.19)

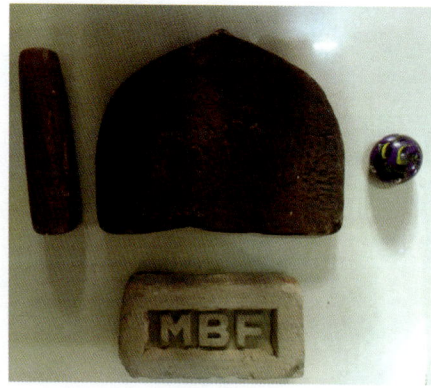

Fig. 4.16: Heavy blunt weapons

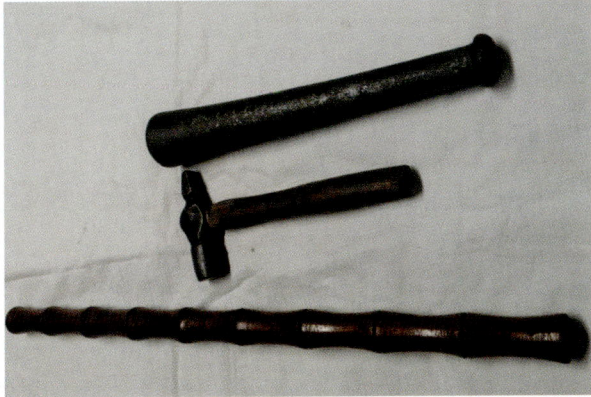

Fig. 4.17: Blunt weapons

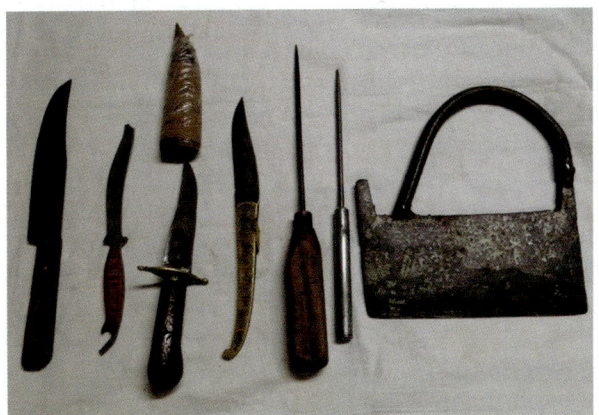

Fig. 4.18: Sharp edged, pointed and heavy cutting weapons

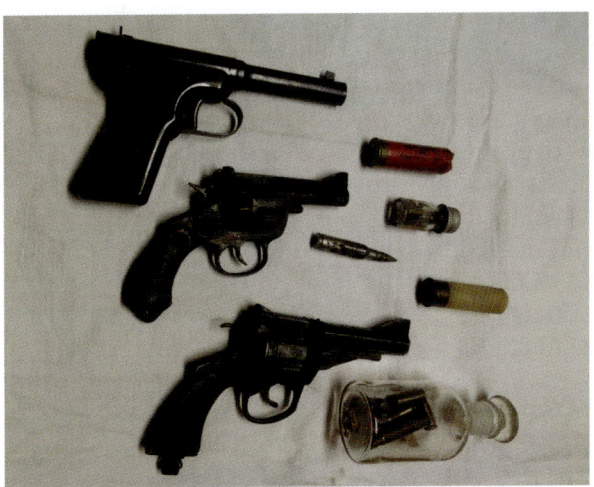

Fig. 4.19: Firearm weapon (pistols, revolver), bullet, pellet and empty cartridge of smooth bore

Age Reporting

Age of an individual is an important aspect for identification. Usually by the order of the court or sometimes the police bring a person to the doctor for estimation of his/her age in a civil or criminal case.

It is important for the doctor to know the medicolegal importance of different ages. The various ages of medicolegal importance are: 1 year, 5 years, 7 years, 10 years, 12 years, 14 years, 17 years, 18 years, 21 years, 25 years, 35 years, 60 years and 65 years.

The following are some of the medicolegal importance of different ages:
1. 1 year and below is the age for framing a charge of infanticide.
2. 7–12 years old child is not held criminally responsible for his act.
3. 12 years old child can give consent for general physical examination and need not take oath in the court.
4. 14 years and above is the age for employment in a factory or for hazardous jobs.
5. 17 years is the minimum age for entrance into a medical/engineering college
6. 18 years old girl can give a valid consent for sex, below that age it is considered rape even if she has given her consent.
7. 18 years is the age of attainment of majority both for girls and boys.
8. 18 years is the minimum age of marriage for a female
9. 21 years is the minimum age of marriage for a male
10. 60 years is the age of retirement from government and many private services.

Time to time there has been various amendments in the age in both civil and criminal cases.

Recently in 2015 the age of consent for sexual intercourse by a female has been raised from 16 to 18 years. Age of retirement for government doctors has been increased from 62 to 65 years. Age estimation of juvenile offenders is the commonest of all age estimation cases brought to the doctor, because in case of offence by teenager the defense lawyer always tries to prove the accused is less than 18 years so that he/she is tried in a juvenile court with significantly less degree of punishment, as happened in the famous Nirbhaya case in Delhi in 2015.

Age of an individual can be determined by the following methods:
1. General physical examination
2. Dental examination
3. Radiological examination

General Physical Examination

It involves measurement of height and weight, voice, secondary sexual characters, hairs over scalp, axilla, chest, moustache and beards (in males), pubic hair, development of genitalia and breast (in females).

Axillary hairs appear by 14–15 years in female and 16–17 years in males. In females pubic hairs are sparse downy, soft and light colored appear by 12–13 years, become thick, dark, curly and bushy by 14–15 years. Pubic hairs appear one year later in males.

Breasts start developing by 12–13 years along with onset of menarche in females.

Tanner staging of puberty should be followed for adolescent age group.

Examination of female subjects should be done by a lady doctor.

Dental Examination

Doctor should be conversant with the difference between deciduous and permanent teeth.

The following should be noted by using a torch in both maxilla and mandible:

1. Teeth erupted or not
2. Type of teeth erupted—deciduous/permanent
3. Space for 3rd molar tooth
4. Missing tooth
5. Any other information

Dental charting as per Palmar/Zsigmondy system as below is usually followed:

a. For primary/deciduous teeth the following dental charting is used:

There are 20 primary teeth which are represented in four quadrants, two each for upper (maxilla) and lower (mandible) jaw as follows.

Upper right (UR)	Upper left (UL)
E D C B A	A B C D E
E D C B A	A B C D E
Lower right (LR)	Lower left (LL)

A = 1st incisor, B = 2nd incisor, C = canine, D = 1st molar, E = 2nd molar

The premolar teeth are absent in the primary/deciduous set of teeth (Figs 5.1 and 5.7)

b. For permanent teeth the following dental charting is used—there are 32 permanent teeth (Fig. 5.5) which are represented as follows.

8 7 6 5 4 3 2 1	1 2 3 4 5 6 7 8
8 7 6 5 4 3 2 1	1 2 3 4 5 6 7 8

1 = 1st incisor, 2 = 2nd incisor, 3 = canine, 4 = 1st premolar, 5 = 2nd premolar, 6 = 1st molar, 7 = 2nd molar, 8 = 3rd molar (Figs 5.2 and 5.8)

Sometimes the 3rd molar may be congenitally absent or the crown is not visible but the root is present. In such cases if required Oral Pan Tomogram (OPG)—a radiological examination of jaw should be advised to see the roots of the teeth (Fig. 5.29).

Age of eruption of temporary and permanent teeth are as follows

Type of teeth	Age of eruption of temporary teeth	Age of eruption of permanent teeth
Lower central incisor	6–7 months	7–8 years
Upper central incisor	7–8 months	7–8 years
Lower lateral incisors	8–9 months	8–9 years
Upper lateral incisors	8–9 months	8–9 years
Canines	18–20 months	11–12 years
First premolars	Absent	9–10 years

Second premolars	Absent	10–11 years
First molar	12 months	6–7 years
Second molar	20–30 months	12–14 years
Third molars	Absent	17–25 years

(Figs 5.1, 5.2, 5.5 and 5.6)

Age of mixed dentition is 6–11 years when both temporary and permanent teeth are present in a child (Figs 5.3 and 5.4).

Dental examination help in assessing the age of a child and adult up to 25 years with fair amount of accuracy.

After the age of 25 years Gustafson's formula is used mostly in dead person.

Radiological Examination

It is one of the most useful tools for estimation of age of an individual as compared to the above two. The doctor should be conversant with the age of appearance and fusion of ossification centers of long bones, appearance of carpal and tarsal bones, sternebrae, sacral vertebrae and closer of skull sutures. Depending on the alleged age, general, physical and dental examination of the following radiographs should be advised:

1. **Wrist joint** for carpal bones, lower ends of radius and ulna (Figs 5.9a and b and 5.10a–c)
2. **Elbow joint** for upper end of radius, ulna, medial and lateral epicondyle of humerus and trochlea of ulna (Figs 5.11a and b)
3. **Shoulder joint** for upper end of humerus and acromion process of scapula (Figs 5.13, 5.17 and 5.18).
4. **Chest** for medial end of clavicle and sternum (Figs 5.14 and 5.18).
5. **Pelvis with hip joint** for ischopubic rami, ischial tuberosity, triradiate cartilage, iliac crest, lesser and greater trochanter of femur (Figs 5.19–5.21).

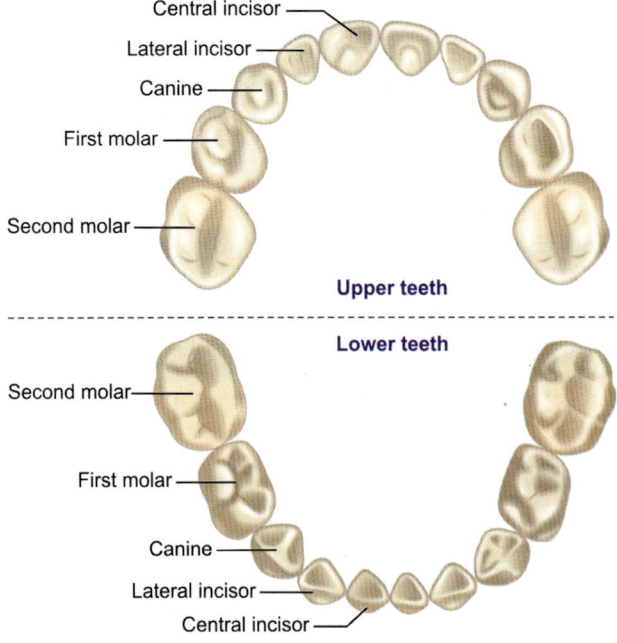

Fig. 5.1: Primary or deciduous teeth

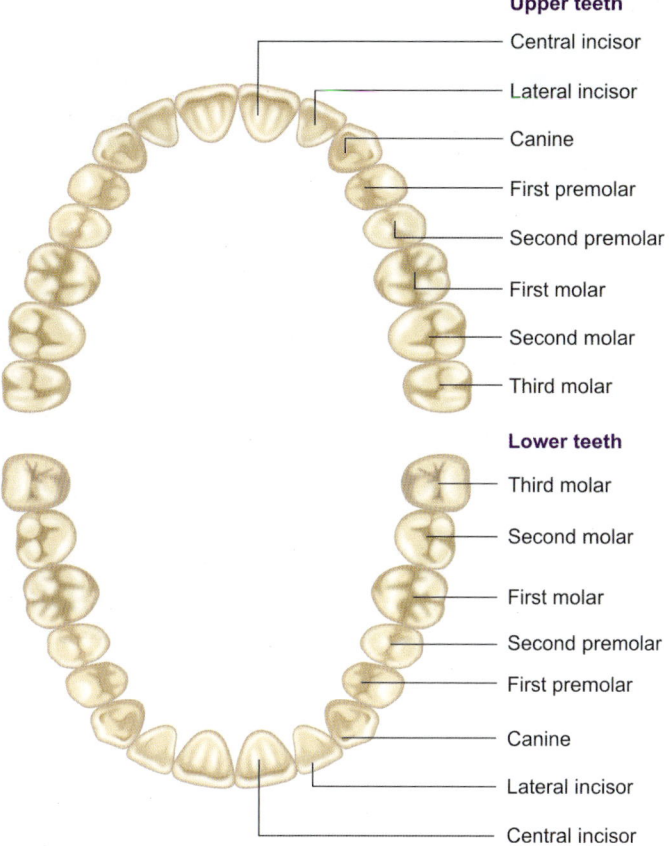

Upper teeth
- Central incisor
- Lateral incisor
- Canine
- First premolar
- Second premolar
- First molar
- Second molar
- Third molar

Lower teeth
- Third molar
- Second molar
- First molar
- Second premolar
- First premolar
- Canine
- Lateral incisor
- Central incisor

Fig. 5.2: Permanent or secondary teeth

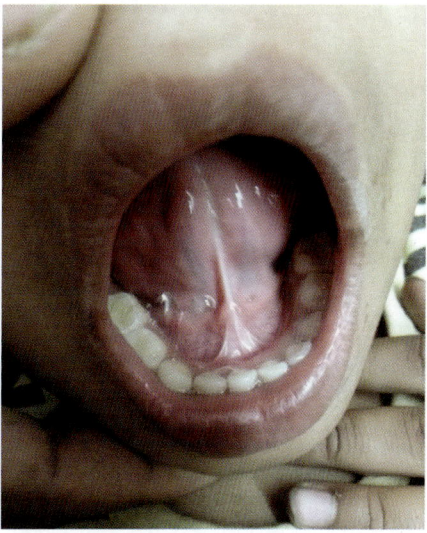

Fig. 5.3: Mixed dentition in a 8-year-old child

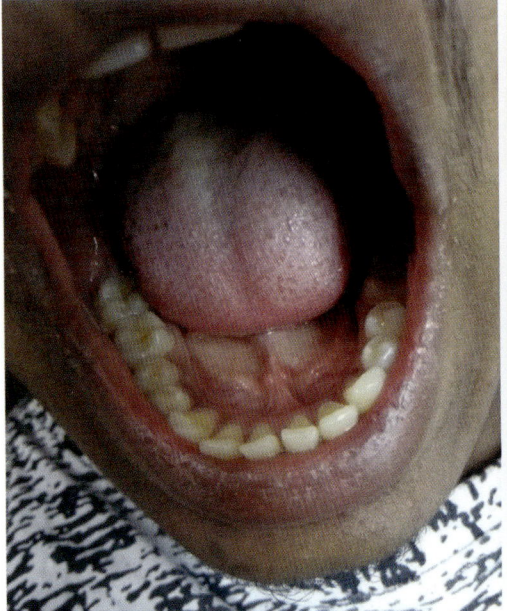

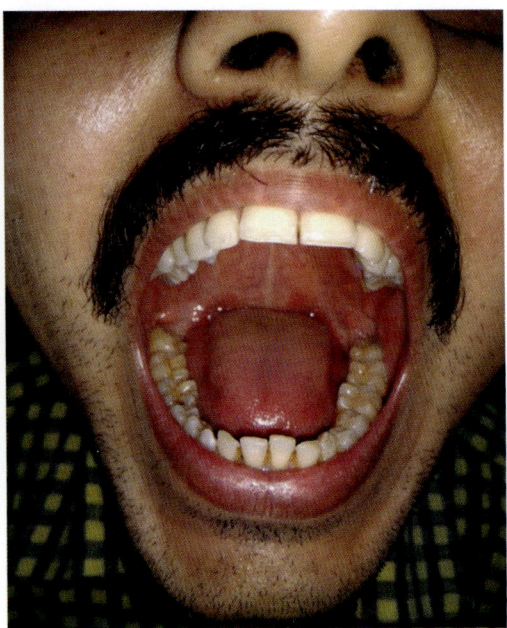

Fig. 5.4: Absence of third molar in a 15-year-old

Fig. 5.5: Presence of all the 16 teeth in the lower jaw including third molar in a 30-year-old

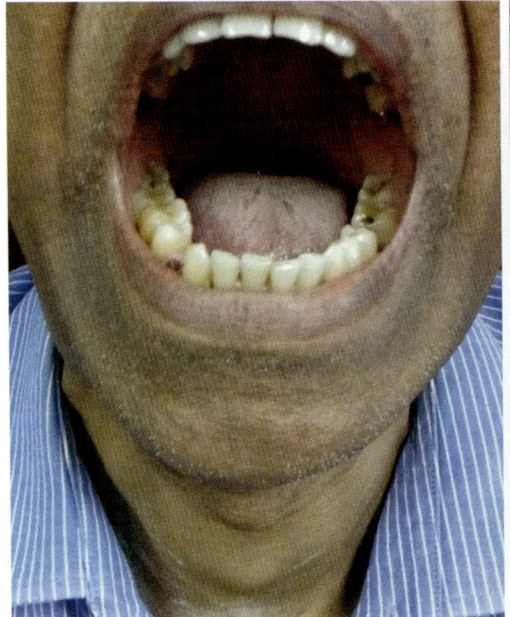

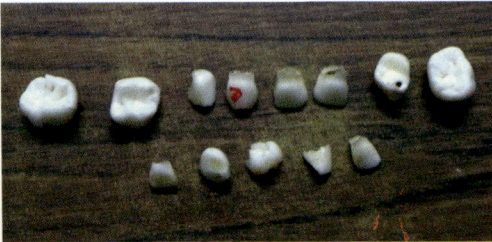

Fig. 5.7: Temporary teeth (isolated)

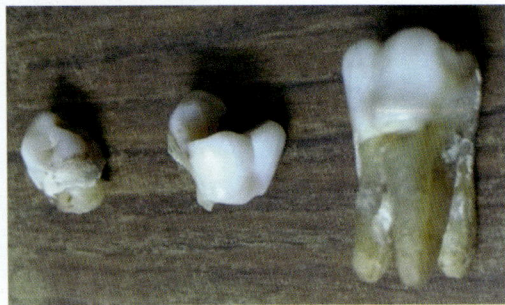

Fig. 5.6: Shedding of first premolar on right side and first molar on left side of lower jaw in a 60-year-old

Fig. 5.8: Permanent tooth: 3rd molar with 3 roots (isolated)

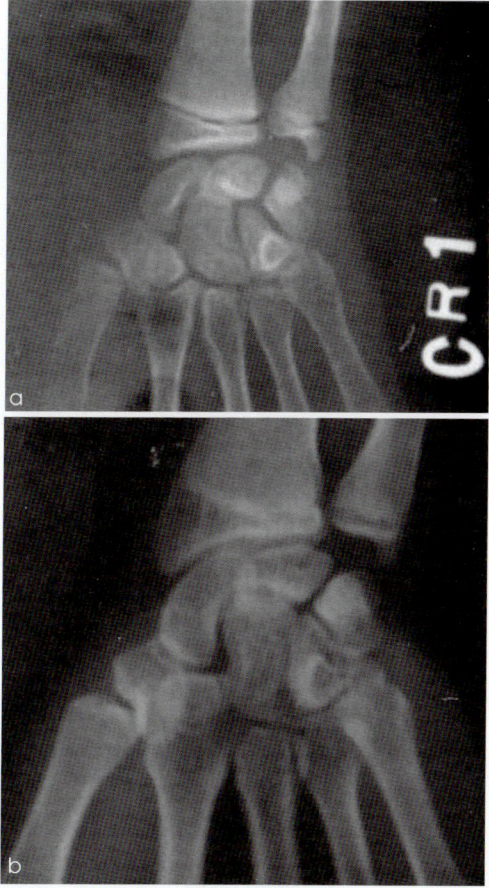

Fig. 5.9: (a) X-ray of non-union at wrist joint; (b) X-ray of complete union at wrist joint

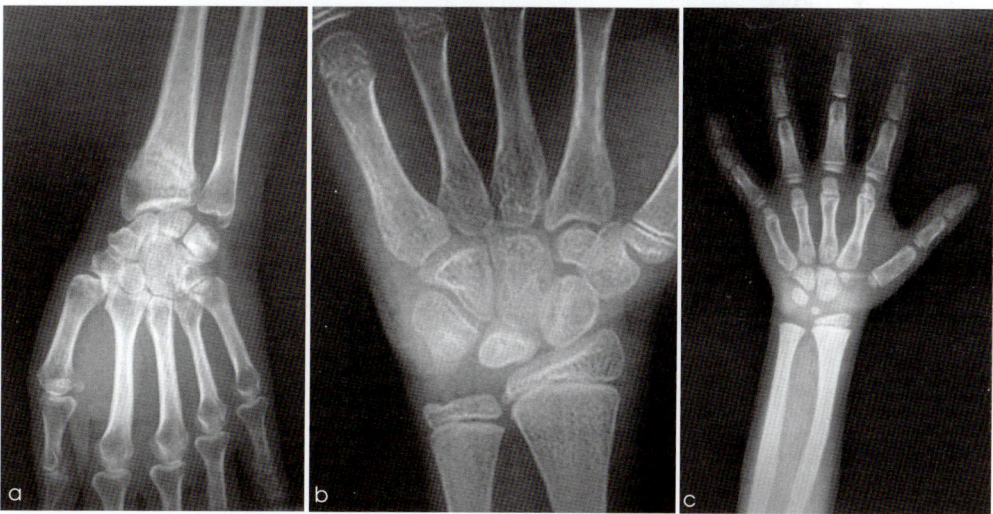

Fig. 5.10: (a) X-ray of wrist joint of 20-year-old person; (b) X-ray of wrist joint of a 14-year-old boy; (c) X-ray of wrist joint of a 6-year-old child

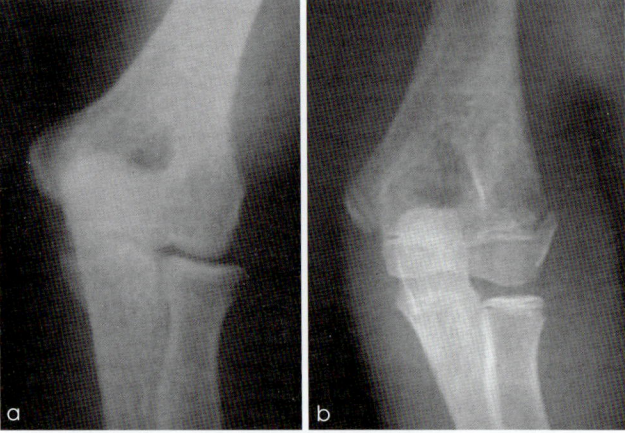

Fig. 5.11: (a) X-ray of complete union at elbow joint; (b) X-ray of non-union at elbow joint

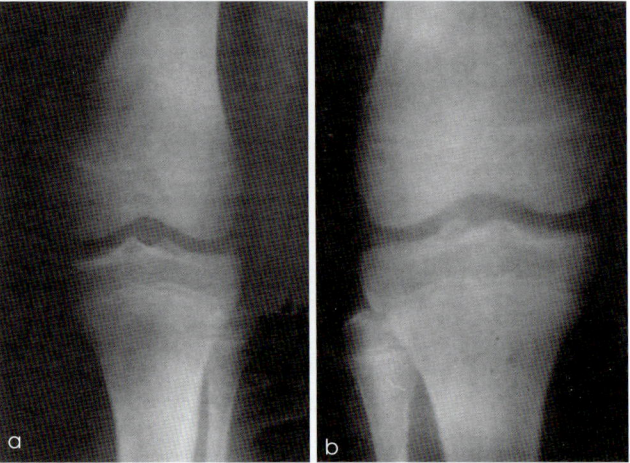

Fig. 5.12: (a) X-ray of complete union at knee joint; (b) X-ray of non-union at knee joint

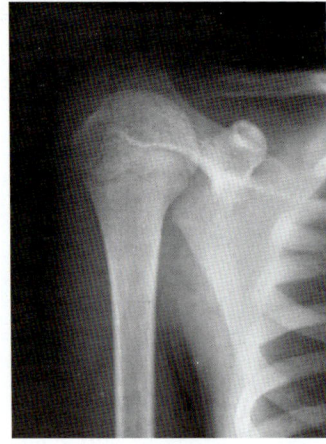

Fig. 5.13: X-ray showing non-union of bones at the upper end of humerus (shoulder joint)

6. **Knee joint** for upper end of tibia, fibula and lower end of femur (Figs 5.12a and b, 5.15, 5.16, 5.22 and 5.23).
7. **Ankle joint** for lower end of tibia, fibula and tarsal bones (Fig. 5.24).
8. **Skull** for saggital, coronal, lambdoid, parietotemporal, basi-occiput sutures.
   Interpretation of the findings on radiographs by a radiologist is desired (Figs 5.25–5.28).

WRIST JOINT

Bones	Appearance	Fusion/Ossification
Lower end of radius	1–2 years	18–19 years
Lower end of ulna	5–6 years	18–19 years
Pisiform		9–12 years
Base of all metacarpals	2–3 years	15–17 years
Head of all metacarpals	1.5–2 years	16–17 years

Wrist joint is completely fused by 18–19 years

ELBOW JOINT

Medial epicondyle of humerus	5–6 years	14–16 years
Lateral epicondyle	11 years	14–16 years
Capitulum	1 year	14–16 years
Trochlea	9–11 years	14–16 years
Head of radius	5–6 years	15–16 years
Head of ulna	8–9 years	16–17 years

Elbow joint is completely fused by 16–17 years

SHOULDER JOINT

Head of humerus	1 year	
Greater tubercle	3 years	4–5 years with head
Lesser tubercle	5 years	
Composite of above three		5–6 years
Composite epiphysis with shaft		17–18 years
Acromion process	14–15 years	17–18 years

Shoulder joint is completely fused by	**17–18 years**	
clavicle medial end	**15–17 years**	**20–22 years**

STERNUM

Bones	Appearance	Fusion/Ossification
1st sternebra	5th month of IU life	25 years with 2nd sternebra
2nd sternebra	7th month of IU life	20 years with 3rd sternebra
3rd sternebra	7th month of IU life	14 years with 4th sternebra
4th sternebra	10th month of IU life	40 years with xiphisternum
Manubrium sternum	5th month of IU life	>60 years with the body
Xiphisternum	3 years after birth	40–50 years with the body

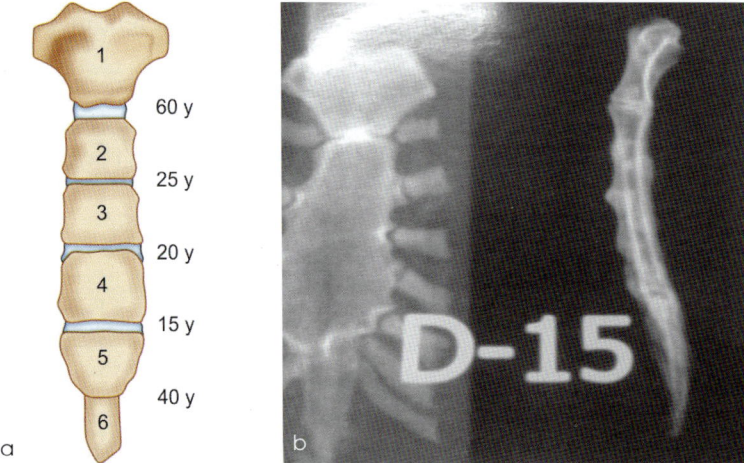

a

b

Fig. 5.14: (a) Sternum showing age of fusion of manubrium, sternebra and xiphisternum; (b) X-ray showing non-union of manubrium with body of sternum, A-P and lateral view

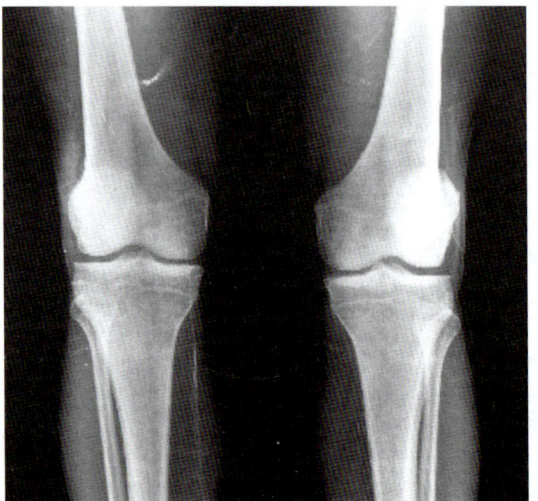

Fig. 5.15: X-ray of complete union at knee joint

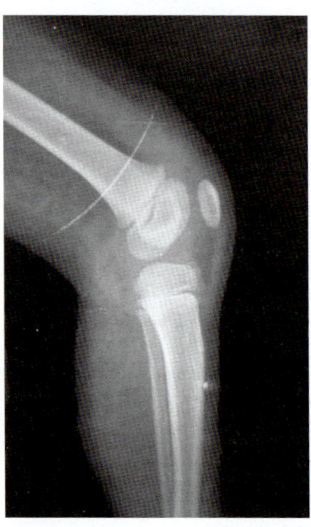

Fig. 5.16: X-ray of non-union at knee joint

PELVIS

Iliac crest	15–16 years	19–21 years
Triradiate cartilage		12–14 years
Ischiopubic rami		7–8 years
Ischial tuberosity	16–17 years	21–22 years

All the bones of pelvis completely fused by 21–22 years

HIP JOINT

Head of femur	1 year	17–18 years with the shaft
Greater trochanter	4 years	14–15 years with the shaft
Lesser trochanter	14 years	15–17 years with the shaft

Hip joint is completely fused by 17–18 years

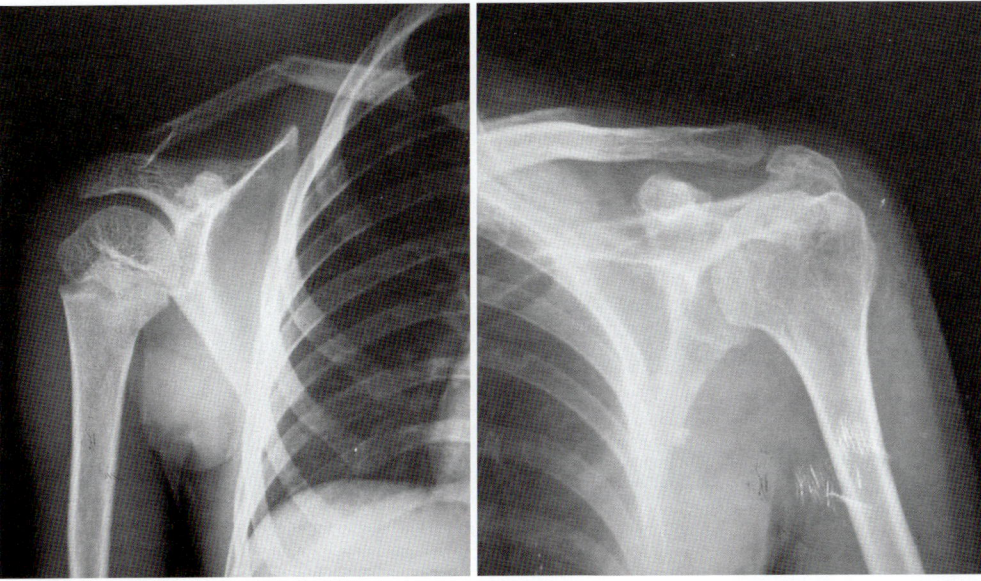

Fig. 5.17: X-ray of non-union at shoulder joint   **Fig. 5.18:** X-ray of complete union at shoulder joint

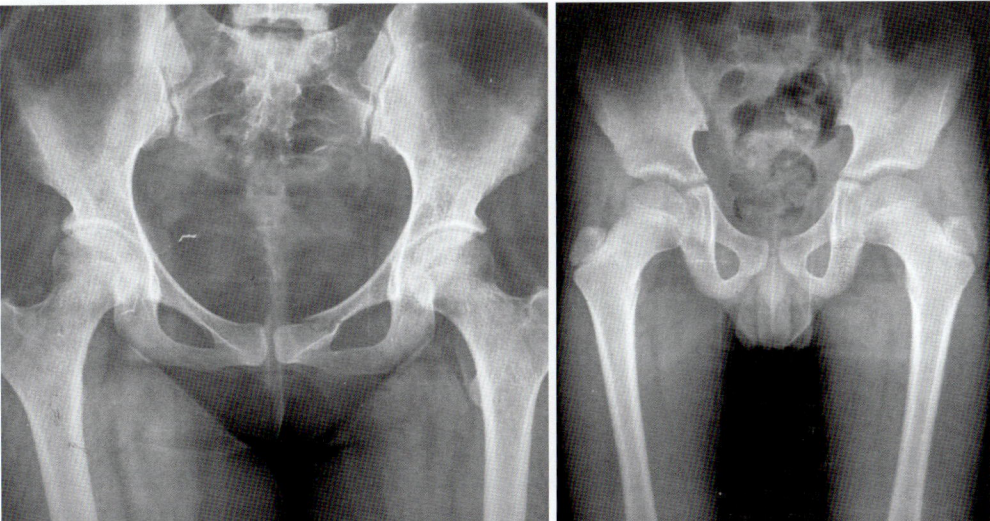

Fig. 5.19: X-ray of complete union of pelvic joint and   **Fig. 5.20:** X-ray of non-union of pelvic joint and
upper end of femur   upper end of femur

KNEE JOINT

Lower end of femur	9th month of IU life	17–18 years
Upper end of tibia	9th month of IU life	17–18 years
Upper end of fibula	4 years after birth	17–18 years

Knee joint is completely fused by 17–18 years

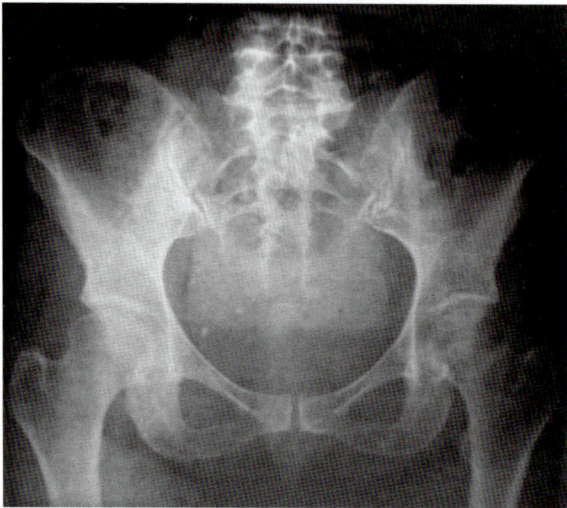

Fig. 5.21: X-ray showing complete union of pelvic bones in a male

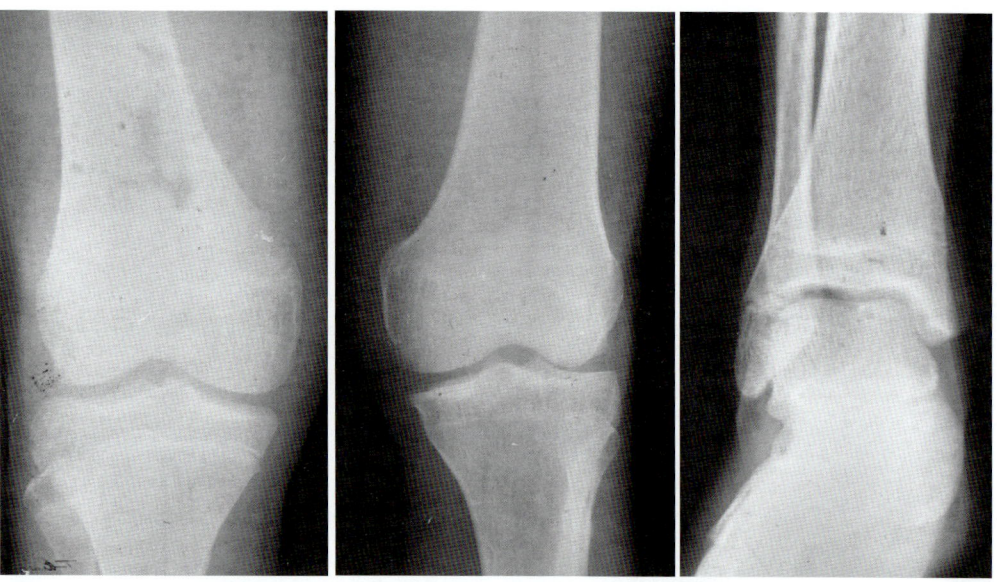

Fig. 5.22: X-ray showing incomplete ossification at knee joint

Fig. 5.23: X-ray showing complete ossification at knee joint

Fig. 5.24: X-ray showing incomplete ossification at ankle joint

ANKLE JOINT

Lower end of tibia	1 year after birth	16–17 years
Lower end of fibula	2 years after birth	16–17 years

Knee joint is completely fused by 16–17 years
Long bone joints unite 1–2 years earlier in females than males

TARSAL BONES

Calcaneum	5th month of IU life
Cuboid	9th month of IU life
Talus	7th month of IU life

SKULL SUTURE

Saggital	25–30 years (posterior one-third), 30–35 years (anterior one-third) and 35–40 years (middle one-third)
Coronal	30–35 years (lower part), 35–40 years (upper part).
Lambdoid	45–50 years
Basiocciput unites with basisphenoid	18–21 years
Metopic (between right and left half of frontal bone)	2–4 years, can extend up to 6 years. May remain unfused in 5% persons.
Parietotemporal	60–70 years
Anterior fontanelle	Closes by 18 months after birth
Posterior fontanelle	Closes by 6–8 months after birth.
Pterion (region of skull where frontal, parietal, temporal and sphenoid join together)	65 years
Asterion (region of skull where lambdoid, parietomastoid and occipitomastoid sutures meet)	50 years

Skull sutures fuse earlier in males than females.

After studying all the radiographs the following columns should be filled up:
Date of X-ray done: ....
Date of X-rays examined: ....
X-ray plate number: ....
Total number of X-ray plates examined: ....
Radiological findings of all the X-ray plates: ....
Age from radiological examination of all the radiographs: ....

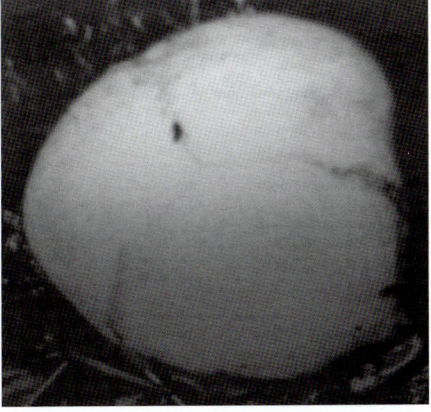

Fig. 5.25: Skull showing non-union of all the sutures

AGE REPORT PROFORMA

CR No. ....   MLC No. ....   Date............................

Name: ....s/o, w/o, d/o...............................Sex........

Addresss...

Referred from.. Brought by (Name of police official/person)..

No. of police official-------Police station-----, Time and place of examination.......................

Age alleged by the person/guardian of the person to be examined....................................

Identification marks:

    1)

    2)

Consent of the person/guardian to be examined..

Name of female attendant/nurse present (in case of female subject)....................................

General physical examination findings..

Age from general physical examination..

Hairs: Axillary, pubic, chest, beard and moustache (in males)

Genitalia type: Child/ adolescent/ adult (in males)

Dental formula...

Age from dental examination...

Radiological examination findings ....

Age from radiological examination ....

Opinion:

    After general physical, dental and radiological examination, I am of the opinion that the age of the subject is between------and-------years.

Signature of Doctor

Name, Designation and Registration No.

(Official Seal of the Doctor)

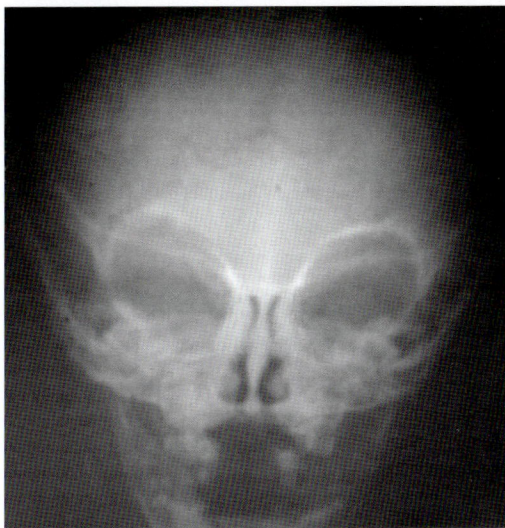

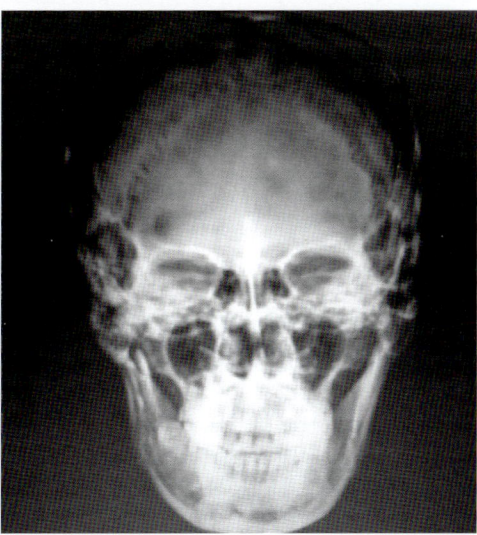

Fig. 5.26: X-ray showing non-union of coronal and sagittal suture

Fig. 5.27: X-ray showing non-union of coronal suture of skull

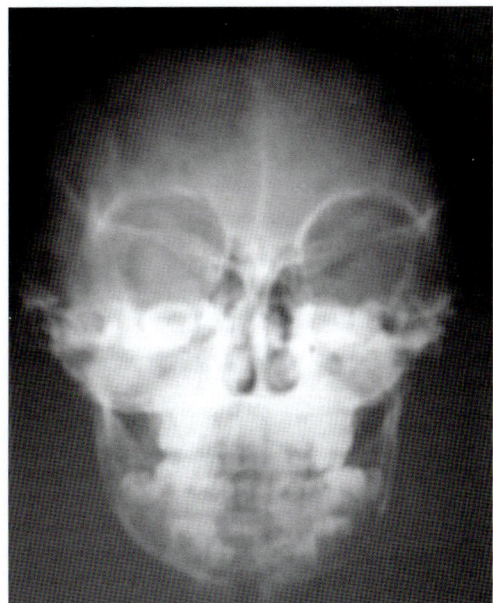

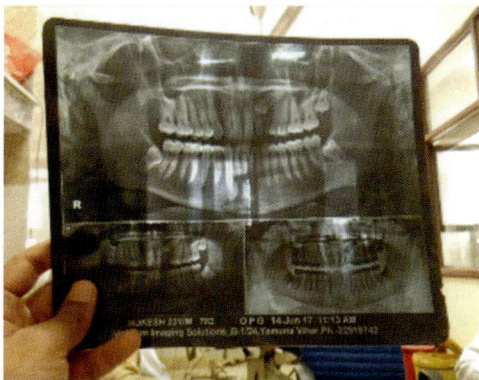

Fig. 5.28: X-ray showing complete union of all the skull sutures

Fig. 5.29: OPG showing impacted 3rd molar tooth

CHAPTER
6

Alcohol/Drunkenness
Case Reporting

Drunkenness is a condition (as defined by British Medical Council in 1927) when the person concerned must be so much under the influence of alcohol, so as to have lost control of his/her faculties to such an extent as to render him/her unable to execute safely the occupation in which he/she was engaged with at the material time.

Practical Aspects about Alcohol

Ethyl alcohol is the commonest form of alcohol from forensic point of view.

It belongs to the inebriant subgroup of cerebral neurotic poison.

Initially in small doses it stimulates the CNS by inhibiting the inhibitory neurons which is responsible for the feeling of well-being, ultimately causing depression of CNS leading to coma and death in heavy doses.

Alcohol is mainly absorbed from the intestines (80%) and from the stomach (20%). About 60% of alcohol is absorbed in the first 60 minutes (Figs 6.1–6.3).

- Fat and proteins delays, while an empty stomach hastens its absorption.
- Alcohol absorption is increased when the concentration is between 10 and 20% and decreased when it is below 10% or above 40% (because of pylorospasm and mucus secretion which delays its flow from stomach to intestines)
- Insulin increases and atropine delays alcohol absorption.
- Absorption increases when taken with carbonated soft drinks (bubbles increase the surface area for absorption)

Alcohol concentration in body fluids after ingestion:
Blood: Urine = 1:1.31
Blood: Exhaled Air = 1:2100
Blood: Saliva = 1:12

Alcohol concentration of blood falls at the rate of 20 mg% per hour

Blood alcohol concentration (BAC) is commonly determined by immunoassay or gas chromatography in the laboratory.

Stages and Symptoms of Alcohol Intoxication based on Blood Alcohol Concentration (BAC)

Remembers 7Ds for 7 stages (Table 6.1).

Medicolegally stages (3) and (4) of alcohol intoxication are the most important as criminal offences are usually committed during these two stages.

Blood alcohol concentration (mg/100 ml)	Stage of intoxication	Symptoms
Table 6.1: Seven stages and symptoms of alcohol intoxication		
0–50	1. Decent/sober	Normal behavior
50–100	2. Delighted/euphoria	Feeling of well-being, overconfident, talkative, disturbed fine movement
100–150	3. Delirious/excited	Memory impairment, unstable emotion and gait
150–200	4. Dazed/confused	Slurred speech, diplopia, disoriented, staggering gait.
200–300	5. Dejected/stupor	Unable to stand, very lethargic, may vomit, decreased response to stimulus.
300–500	6. Dead drunk/coma	Looses consciousness, no response to stimuli, incontinence, laboured breathing.
>500	7. Death	Respiratory failure leading to death

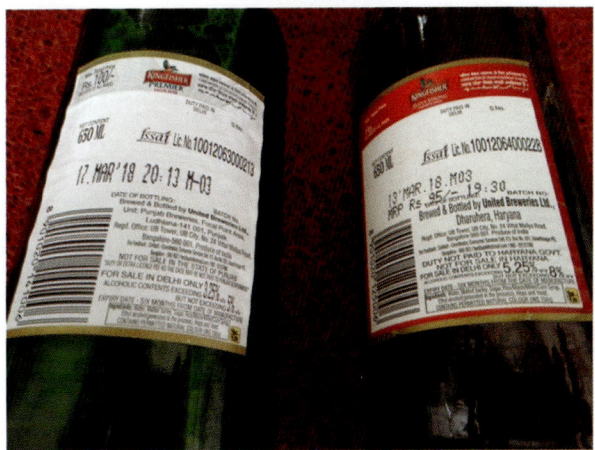

Fig. 6.1: Alcohol—beer with alcohol content of 3.25% and 5.25%

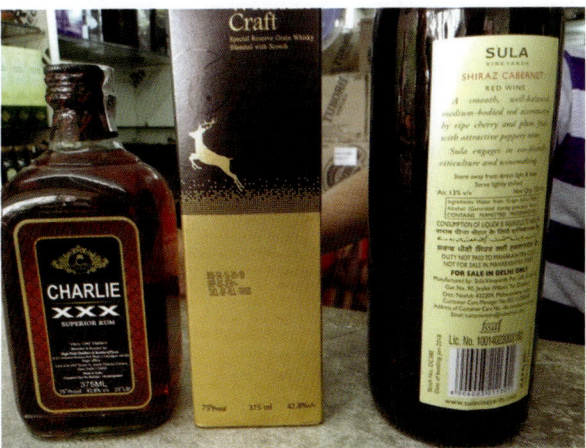

Fig. 6.2: Alcohol—rum, whisky and wine with alcohol content of 42.8%

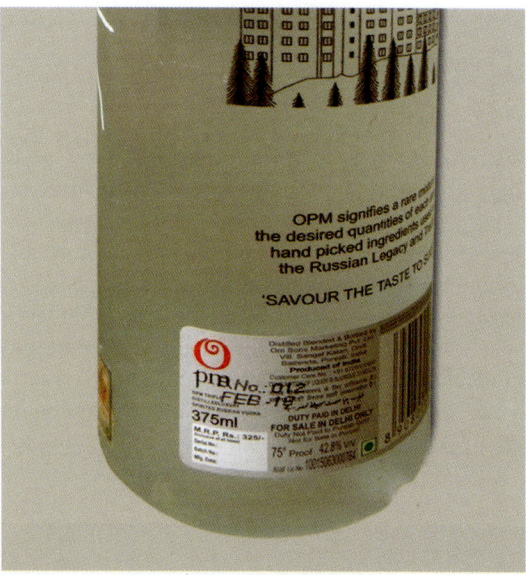

Fig. 6.3: Alcohol—vodka with alcohol content of 42.8%

Delirium tremens is a condition of mind seen in chronic alcoholics due to
1. Sudden withdrawal of alcohol (for 3–5 days)
2. Excessive intake of alcohol
3. Receiving severe injury leading to shock
4. Acute infection

Signs and symptoms of delirium tremens:
1. Coarse muscular tremors of face, tongue and hands
2. Restlessness, agitation, insomnia, memory loss
3. Suicidal, homicidal or violent assault tendency
4. Hallucination—visual and auditory
5. Disoriented to time and space
6. Level of consciousness effected

Medicolegal Importance of Drunkenness

1. Alcohol consumption is an offence in states where there exists a Prohibition Act, e.g. Gujarat, Bihar, Nagaland and Lakshadweep and some districts of Manipur.
2. In traffic accidents both the driver of the vehicle (under the Motor Vehicle Act, 1988) and the victim are examined for alcohol intake to fix the liability of the accident. In India the statutory limit of blood alcohol is 30 mg% for safe driving.
3. Voluntary drunken person is responsible for a crime (under Section 86 IPC), unless the alcohol was administered to him without his knowledge or against his will (under Section 85 IPC)
4. A drunken person's consent is not considered valid.
5. A doctor in a drunken state should not attend and treat a person. If the doctor does so he/she can be sued for professional misconduct with penal eraser of his/her name from the state register if some physical damage is caused to the patient.

6. A surgeon can be charged for Rash and Negligent Act (under Section 304A of IPC) if the patient dies during surgery, if the surgeon in a drunken state performed an operation.

7. Misconduct by a drunken person in public is punishable under Section 510 IPC with 24 hours imprisonment.

8. A drunken person cannot make a valid Will.

9. Drinking in public places and near liquor shops in Delhi will attract a fine up to Rs. 10,000/and a jail term for 3 months under the Delhi Excise Act from 7th November, 2016. However, the matter is debatable.

10. If a drunken person is under the custody of a police and refuses consent, then the doctor can proceed with the examination even without the consent using a reasonable degree of force under Section 53(1), CrPC.

11. Under Section 84 IPC a person under Delirium Tremens is not held liable for any crime because of unsoundness of mind.

12. The legal age for drinking in India varies from state to state ranging between 18 and 25 years.

Proforma For Examination of A Case of Drunkenness

CR No. ....   MLC No. ....   Date...........................

Name...S/D/W of.............................

Age.............Sex...............,Religion..................,Residential Address...........................

Occupation............., Brought by (Name, address of relative or friend) ....

Name and no. of investigating officer .... Police Station ....

Date, time and place of examination ....

Identification marks:

    1.

    2.

Informed consent (if possible): As above in injury and age reporting, additionally for collection of blood and urine samples. If subject is not in a position for consent, next of the kin can give consent.

Brief History of the Case

- Whether or not the subject has consumed alcohol.
- If consumed, quantity, type (whisky/rum/bear/local made, etc.) and time of consumption.
- Whether used to taking alcohol
- What was the time of last food intake or consumed
- Whether suffering from any medical illness and on medication
- Which medicines were taken before consuming alcohol?

General and Physical Examination

- **Clothes** for presence of vomitus, salivary stains, soiled or not.
- **Breath** smells of alcohol, tongue furred, dry or moist

- **Pulse** is rapid (should be checked at the beginning and end of examination).
- **Temperature** may be subnormal or raised
- **Face** is flushed or not
- **Eyelids** swollen and conjunctiva congested or not
- **Pupils** dilated/constricted and pupillary reaction time.
- **McEvans** sign is positive when a constricted pupil becomes dilated after pinching or slapping on face followed by a very slow return to constricted state. Whether it is positive or not.
- **Alcohol gaze nystagmus (AGN)** is an involuntary jerky movement of the eyes as they gaze to the sides. It can be tested by asking the subject to gaze at your finger while moving it from the center of his/her face to both the sides. It is usually seen at **blood alcohol concentration (BAC) of 80–100 mg/100 ml**, whether it is positive or not.
- AGN is because of the effect of alcohol on the vestibulo-cochlear system.
- Behavior is aggressive, abusive or submissive
- Memory and mental alertness are diminished or not which can be tested by asking the time, date and to solve simple addition and subtraction. There could also be loss of judgement.
- Speech is slurred and thick or normal, blurring of certain words is an early sign of incoordination, which is confirmed by asking the subject to pronounce some words/sentence.
- Fine movements of fingers with tremors are present or not which can be tested by asking him/her to write any sentence and observing omission or repetition of words or letters. **Features of incoordination are seen when BAC is between 150 and 200 mg/100 ml.**
- Gait is staggering or not. The person is asked to walk nine steps heel-to-toe in a straight line and then turn and come back. Observe if he/she steps off the line, stops or uses hands to maintain balance, number of steps are incorrect. **If the above signs are positive, the BAC is around 80%.**
- Romberg's test—the person is asked to stand with the feet together and eyes closed. If the person sways or falls, the test is considered positive. The observer should stand close to the subject to prevent him/her from sustaining any injury due to fall.

Muscle Coordination Tests

- *Finger nose test:* The person is asked to touch the tip of nose by an outstretched hand with eyes closed. If unable to perform, coordination is impaired.
- **Buttoning and unbuttoning a shirt** can perform or not.
- **Picking up some objects from floor** can perform or not.
- **Lighting up cigarette with matchstick** can perform or not.
- **Reflexes**
  - Knee and ankle reflexes are sluggish
  - Plantar reflex is flexor or extensor
  - Must rule out any CNS disease before performing the above tests.

Collection of Samples

1. **Blood** should be collected from antecubital or femoral vein. The skin should be cleaned using soap water or 1:1000 solution of mercuric chloride (should not use surgical spirit as it contains alcohol). About 5 ml of blood should be collected.

   The preservative used is 50 mg of sodium fluoride for 5 ml blood in a glass bottle. The bottle is thoroughly shaken and closed with a tight stopper sealed with paraffin wax.

   This prevents loss of alcohol by glycolysis and bacterial action.

2. **Urine** should be collected the whole amount that is passed at the time. The preservative is sodium chloride or thymol.

3. **Breath:** The person should be asked to blow into a breath analyser or alcometer. This is usually used by traffic police or casualty of a hospital for immediate result.

Opinion

After detailed examination the opinion should be given as—I am of the opinion that the person

1. Has not consumed alcohol.
2. Has consumed alcohol but is not under the influence of it.
3. Has consumed alcohol and is under its influence.

Signature of the Doctor
Name, Designation and Registration No.
Official Seal of the Doctor

Sexual Offence Case Reporting

Sexual offence is defined as illegal sexual act done by one person with another or with animal.

It can be classified as:

1. **Natural** which involves the use of the sexual organs meant for normal sexual intercourse (peno-vaginal), viz.
   a. Rape
   b. Incest
   c. Adultery
2. **Unnatural,** which involves use of organs or parts of body not normally meant for sexual intercourse, viz
   a. Sodomy (anal coitus)
   b. Buccal (oral) coitus
   c. Lesbianism (sexual relations between two females)
3. **Sexual perversions** in which sexual gratification is obtained by acts totally unrelated to sex, viz
   a. Sadism
   b. Masochism
   c. Fetishism, etc.

Majority of the sexual perversions are not considered as sexual offence as the person involved is suffering from one or the other mental illness and does not enjoy the normal sexual activity. However, this can lead to marital disharmony and divorce.

- Masturbation in public is an obscene act if done in public in front of a woman. It is punishable under IPC Section 354 (outraging the modesty of a woman) and IPC Section 509 (gestures and acts intended to insult and outrage the modesty of a female).
- After the recent amendments in criminal law, the age of consent for sexual intercourse of female has been raised from 16 to 18 years.
- Punishment for the offence in aggravated situation has been enhanced from 7 years to rigorous imprisonment for 10 years which may extend to life imprisonment.
- **In case the rape victim dies or remains in persistent vegetative state, the accused** shall be punished with rigorous imprisonment for 20 years which may extend to life imprisonment which means the natural life, the accused will bear the medical expenses and rehabilitation of the victim as per new Section 376A IPC.
- Police requisition/FIR is not mandatory for seeking medical care and treatment of an alleged rape victim.

The cases of sexual offence commonly encountered are rape and sodomy.

In both the cases both the victim as well as the accused should be examined to arrive at a final opinion. An alleged victim of rape should be examined by a registered lady doctor from the department of obstetrics and gynaecology. The victim should be received with a sympathetic and sensitive attitude by the medical team.

Proforma For Examination Of An Alleged Rape Victim

CR No. .... MLC No.............................. Date...........................

Name...

D/W of.., Age................,Religion................

Residential Address... Occupation...............................

Brought by Police Officer, Name..

No. of Police Officer..Police Station......................................

Name and address of accompanying persons and their relationship with the victim...Date, time and place of

examination..Marital status of the victim...........................

Number of children if married............................History alleged by the police

....

History alleged by the victim/ relatives...

Informed Consent: As in any other medicolegal report. She should be informed and explained about the details of her examination and, that she is free to refuse to be examined. In case of minor girl/mentally challenged victim, the consent should be obtained from parents/guardian. Husband has no role in the consent of a married victim.

Identification marks:

1. ....

2. ....

Name of the female attendant/Nurse...

Brief history of the case regarding the following should be asked from the victim:

1. Date, time and place of the incident
2. Was the penetration vaginal, oral or anal
3. Was she in her menstrual phase.
4. Did she struggle and cry for help
5. Was she conscious during the act
6. Was she drugged before the act
7. Is she wearing the same clothes as at the time of the incident or changed.
8. Has she taken bath and cleaned her genitalia after the incident or not.
9. Did she urinate after the sexual assault
10. Total number of accused persons

Examination of the Victim

It should be done at the earliest to avoid loss of any material evidence.

A. General: The following should be observed and recorded:

   a. Degree of mental stress should be assessed and she should be reassured about the importance of her examination

b. Height, weight and built

c. BP and pulse

d. Gait is painful or not

e. Clothes and undergarments are in disarray or not, torn, missing buttons, any stains

f. She should be asked to stand on a large white sheet of paper and undress herself. Any material that falls on the sheet should be collected and preserved.

g. **Extragenital injury** marks in the form of bruise, abrasion laceration on the body as including the inner part of thigh and defence wounds should be noted.

   Love bite marks in the form of discoid bruises caused by sucking kisses of the accused on the skin over breasts and other body parts of the female victim. Extragenital injuries will be absent or minimum if the victim is a child, mentally challenged or intoxicated adult as they are unable to offer resistance to the sexual assault.

   Some extra genital injuries will be present in a virgin. Maximum extra genital injuries will be present in a deflorated woman (who is used to sexual intercourse) as she will offer maximum resistance during sexual assault.

h. Fingernail if broken or not, any foreign material in the nailbed should be looked for and collected by scrapping it and preserved. It is done to confirm the dried blood and epithelial cells/soft tissues of the alleged accused.

i. Breasts should be looked for bite marks, bruise and abrasions caused by the alleged accused.

B. **Genital:** The female should be examined in lithotomy position under sufficient illumination.

   a. The pubic hair should be looked for any matting due to dried seminal discharge of the accused. The matted hair should be cut and put in an envelope and send for matching of the semen with that of the alleged accused.

   b. The pubic hair of the female should be combed on a white sheet of paper to look for any male pubic hair which is put in an envelope and send to be compared with that of the alleged accused.

   c. The vulva, introitus, vagina, perineum and anus should be looked for inflammation, fingernail marks and bleeding. Invisible injuries can be visualized by using colposcopy which is a binocular microscope on wheels with up to 30 times magnification and illumination.

   d. Genital injuries are extensive and severe when she is a child because of the disproportion between the size of the adult penis and small vagina. Since the hymen is deeply situated in a child it is not usually ruptured.

   e. Genital injuries in adult virgin is common even if it is done with her consent. The hymen will be ruptured if there is full penetration of penis.

   f. Genital injuries are a few or absent when she is a married female and used to sexual intercourse. An old healed ruptured hymen is usually seen. Hymenal opening is usually measured by Glaister-keene glass or plastic rods, wooden conical graduated rod or hymenoscope.

   g. Dried or moist seminal stain in and around vagina and inner part of thigh should be looked for.

C. **Anal:** Anus should be examined for tenderness, bruise, abrasion, nail marks, tear laceration over the perianal area and anal mucosa. Perineal tear if any should be examined. The subject should be examined in knee-elbow position. A labeled anatomical diagrammatic clockwise representation should be made of the above findings.

Sample Collection

The following samples should be collected, duly sealed with the seal of the doctor and sent to CFSL through the IO of the case.
1. Clothes are dried and made into a parcel.
2. Vaginal swabs low and high (up to cervix) for semen.
3. Vaginal washings after irrigation with normal saline for semen.
4. Pubic hair (if present) both matted and combed.
5. Finger nails scrapping.
6. Blood for DNA profiling and sexually transmitted diseases.
7. Semen containing intact spermatozoa for DNA typing
8. Salivary stains swabs from the kissed parts of the female body for secretor status of the accused
9. Swabs from oral cavity including pharynx in oral and from rectum in anal coitus.
10. Urine for presence of spermatozoa
11. Any other foreign material or trace evidence like mud, grass leaves that will indicate the place of the crime.

SAFE (Sexual Assault Forensic Evidence) Kit

The physical evidence of samples collected as above by the doctor in case an alleged sexual assault is called a SAFE kit or rape kit.
The following articles are present in SAFE kits:
1. A few envelopes for collection of nail scrapings, hair, stains and trace evidences.
2. Tapered wooden sticks for collection of nail scrapings
3. Comb
4. Boxes and glass slides for vaginal, rectal and oral swab collection.
5. Glass vials for collection of blood and vaginal discharge, if any.
6. A clean towel

Opinion

Since rape is a legal definition the doctor should never opine whether rape has been done with a female on the basis of examination findings.
However, if the female victim less than 18 years (age of consent for sex) and on examination by the doctor there is enough evidence of forceful sexual assault on the victim, rape can be said to have been committed.
The opinion is given as follows:
1. There is evidence of recent sexual intercourse if the above genital and extra genital injuries are present along with complete motile spermatozoa (which is found in the vagina for 24 hours, rarely up to 3 days, with passage of time they become non-motile and disintegrate. But can be found up to 2 weeks in endocervix).

2. There is evidence of recent penetration if genital and extragenital injuries are present on the female without any spermatozoa.
3. There is no evidence of penetration when there are no genital or extragenital injuries on her body and no spermatozoa.
4. There is evidence of application of mouth can be judged only if salivary stains of the accused are found over her genitalia/anus
5. There is evidence of touching her genitalia/anus only if finger nail marks /finger prints of the accused are present.

Similar opinion is given in forceful oral and anal coitus depending upon the examination findings.

Signature of the Doctor
Name, designation and registration number
Official Seal of the Doctor

EXAMINATION OF THE ACCUSED

The alleged accused when apprehended for a sexual assault should be examined to prove or disprove his involvement in the crime. It is not uncommon to falsely implicate an innocent male in sexual assault by a female with some ulterious motive against him. Preferably the same doctor as the victim should examine the accused for better correlation. The proforma of examination is the same as for the victim.

Proforma For Examination Of Accused Of Alleged Rape

CR No. .... MLC No............................. Date.........................
Name.., S/o...
Age............, Religion...................., Residential Address..
Occupation.........................., Brought by public............................. or police...................
Name and no. of police officer...........................Police Station..
Date and time of examination...
Identification marks:
1. ....
2. ....

Informed consent: As above in injury and age reporting. He should be told that he is free to refuse being examined. If under police custody doctor can examine even if the subject refuses to give consent by using a reasonable amount of force under Section 53A Cr.PC.
Presence of any attendant is not necessary during the examination.
Brief history given by the police..
Brief history given by the alleged male ....

General Examination

1. Behavior pattern—fearful, aggressive, shy, guilty looking
2. Clothes—ask whether wearing the same clothes or changed. Look for blood stains,

seminal stains, cosmetic stains. Torn with missing buttons or not. Underwear for any stain or tear.
3. Height, weight and build
4. Look for any injury marks on the body likely to be caused by resistance from the female.

Genital Examination

1. Pubic hairs are matted or not
2. Comb the pubic hair for presence of female pubic hair, if any.
3. Genital development—adolescent or adult type.
4. Abrasion, bruise or laceration to the shaft of penis, prepuce, glance and scrotum.
5. Look for smegma under the foreskin of glance penis. Its presence all around indicates there has not been any sexual intercourse with full penetration into vagina for about 24 hours.
6. **Iodine test:** The penis is cleaned with a filter paper. The filter paper is then exposed to vapors of Lugol's iodine. The paper turns brown if vaginal epithelial cells are present on the glans because of the glycogen present in the vaginal cells. This test is positive up to 72–96 hours.
7. **Papanicolaou's test:** After washing the penis with normal saline the washing is stained with Papanicolaou's stain. It will stain the vaginal cells if present indicating penile penetration into the vagina.

Samples Collection

1. Clothes including the underwear
2. Pubic hair and combed hair
3. Blood

Opinion

1. There is nothing to suggest that male subject performed recent sexual intercourse if all the above findings are absent and a thick coating of smegma is present underneath the foreskin of the glance penis.
2. The male subject was involved in recent sexual intercourse if the above findings are present along with positive test result.

Signature of the Doctor
Name, designation and registration number

SODOMY CASE REPORTING

Sodomy is anal intercourse between either two males or between a male and a female. Section 377 IPC deals with the offence of unnatural sexual offence which states that whoever voluntarily has carnal intercourse against the order of nature with a man, woman (non-consensual) or animal, shall be punished with imprisonment of either description for a term which may extend to 10 years and shall be liable to fine. Penetration is sufficient to constitute the carnal intercourse necessary to the offence described in this section.

The section was decriminalized with respect to sex between two consenting adults by the Delhi High Court in July 2009. Supreme Court of India in December 2013 repealed the judgement on Section 377 stating that the matter should be left to the Parliament and not judiciary. On 6th February, 2016 the final hearing of the curative petition filed by Naz Foundation and others is pending in the Supreme Court because of the controversy on the issue of rights raised particularly by LGBT (lesbian, gay, bisexual and transgender) community.

Sodomy involves an active and a passive agent. Consent of passive agent is not a defence and will be punished along with active agent. Sodomite is a person/s, who practice anal intercourse, both active and passive agents. Catamite is a child passive agent.

Examination of a case of sodomy: It involves both examination of victim (passive agent) and accused (active agent).

Proforma For Examination of Passive Agent of Sodomy

CR No .... MLC No .... Date ....
Name ...., S/o ....,
Age ...., Religion ...., Residential ....
Address............ Occupation ...., Brought by police ....
Name and No. of Police officer ....Police station ....
Date and time of examination ....

Identification Marks

1. ....
2. ....

Informed Consent: As in other MLC cases above.
Brief history of the case:
1. Date, time and place
2. Position of passive agent during the act.
3. If lubricant was used by the active agent.
4. Whether wearing the same clothes or changed
5. Whether taken bath and cleaned the anal area.
6. Has defecated after the incident or not.
7. If already suffering from piles, fissures or fistula.

The following should be looked for:
General:
1. Gait—broad based and painful or normal
2. Clothes—torn, stains or loose pubic hair
3. Injury marks over body.

Anal: Examination should be done in knee-elbow position
1. Any tenderness during examination
2. Presence of any lubricant in and around anus
3. Bruise, abrasion or laceration in and around anus

4. Active bleeding or dried blood stains around anus
5. Fresh or dried seminal stains.
6. Anal swab should be collected before internal examination of anus to examine for semen.
7. Per rectal (PR) digital examination for the tone of sphincter ani. Normally it easily admits only one index finger without any discomfort. If two fingers are admitted with feeling of tenderness, full penetration is likely.
8. Proctoscopy examination for visualization of anal and lower rectal mucosal injury.
9. If the victim is a child, extensive laceration of anus and perineum is common finding with blood stains or active bleeding.

In Habitual Passive Agent

1. Anal hair will be shaved
2. Thickened perianal skin
3. Anal orifice is dilated, lax sphincter with absence of anal reflex (contraction of sphincter ani on pinching the anal skin)
4. No tenderness on digital examination and absence of rugae of anal mucosa.
5. The anus may be funnel shaped.
6. Sexually transmitted disease in the form of anal condyloma may be observed.

Opinion

Depending upon the above examination findings and presence of seminal stains.
1. Anal intercourse has been done with the victim.
2. Anal intercourse has not been done with the victim.

Proforma For Examination of Active Agent of Sodomy

CR No. .... MLC No............................. Date ....
Name.., S/o ....,
Age................., Religion ...., Residential ....
Address............ Occupation ...., Brought by police ....
Name and no. of Police officer .... Police station ....
Date and time of examination ....

Identification marks

1. ....
2. ....

Informed consent

As in other MLC cases above. Section 53 A Cr.Pc as above will be applicable in case the accused refuses to give consent.
    The following should be examined:

General

1. Clothes torn or not, presence of any stains
2. Any injury marks on the body produced during struggle with the passive agent.

Penile

1. Bruise, abrasion of prepuce and glance penis
2. Tear of frenulum.
3. Fecal stains or lubricant traces

Opinion about active agent

1. The alleged male was not involved in anal intercourse.
2. The possibility of the alleged male being involved in anal intercourse cannot be ruled out.

Impotency
Case Reporting

Impotency is the inability of a person to perform the act of sexual intercourse. This inability is usually seen in males where there is failure of erection of penis during sexual intercourse and is called erectile dysfunction (ED).

Causes of Impotency in Male

1. Psychological
2. Below the age of puberty, i.e. 14–15 years
3. Hypospadias with chordee
4. Large hydrocoele.
5. Paraplegia
6. Tumor of penis
7. Diabetes
8. Impotence quoad hoc—the male is impotent with a particular female but not with other.

Female Impotency

Although female is a passive partner but plays an active role in arousal leading to erection, penetration and ejaculation of male organ. However, in cases of vaginismus (involuntary contraction of vaginal muscles before the act of sex) and dyspareunia (severe pain during the act of sex) penetration of male organ is not possible. Also when she does not take any interest in sexual activity, a condition called frigidity. These cases are known as female impotency.

Medicolegal Issues

In civil cases:

a. Nullity of marriage
b. Disputed paternity

In criminal cases:

a. Rape
b. Sodomy
c. Buccal coitus.

Proforma for Examination of Case of an Impotency

CR No. .... MLC No............................. Date.........................
Name ...., S/o ....
Age ...., Religion................................, Residential...
Address .... Occupation................ , Brought by police..
Name and no. of police officer .... Police station...
Date and time of examination ....

Identification marks:

1. ....   2. ....

History of any systemic disease like diabetes, drug addiction, psychological illness, any trauma to lower lumbar vertebrae.

Informed consent: As above in injury and age reporting. He should be told that he is free to refuse being examined.

General examination: Height, weight, build and voice.

Local examination

1. Pubic hair present/absent, adolescent/adult type.
2. Penis normal/circumcised/diseased, child/adolescent/adult type.

Tests of Potency

1. **Nocturnal penile tumescence (NPT) test:** In a normal male on an average there are 5–6 penile erections during REM sleep. Its absence indicates some defect in innervation and vascular supply of penis. It helps to distinguish organic from psychogenic cause of ED.
   a. **Snap gauge test:** A ring-shaped device made of plastic film is fitted around the penis. With erection of penis it breaks. It is repeated for 2–3 nights.
   b. **Stamp test:** The penis is wrapped with 1 inch strip of paper all round the shaft. Then stamps are tightly fitted on it. Erection of penis will torn the stamps.
2. **Penile Doppler ultrasound:** This test is used to measure the blood flow of penis using an ultrasound after injecting a combination of papaverine and PGE1 that cause penile erection. Any vascular abnormality causing ED can be diagnosed.
3. **Penile biothesiometry:** It evaluates the nervous sensitivity of the glance penis. It is a measurement of the vibratory sense of the penis using an electromagnetic device.

The potency tests are carried out by a team of doctors consisting of a urologist, radiologist and a psychiatrist.

Opinion

1. There is nothing to suggest that the male is incapable of sexual intercourse, if after examination no abnormality is found.
2. If some gross organic abnormality as listed above is detected, then it should be opined that the male is incapable of sexual intercourse.
3. Although not common the opinion about female impotency should be given with caution, unless there is gross deformity.

Signature of the Doctor
Name, designation, registration number
Official seal of the Doctor

Postmortem Examination—General

Autopsy/necropsy/postmortem examination/thanatopsy are synonyms and deals with the examination of human body for the purpose of investigation after death.

The autopsy can be performed by any registered MBBS doctor posted in a government hospital. However, a doctor having a recognized postgraduate (MD) degree in forensic medicine or pursuing MD forensic medicine from a recognized medical college with postmortem facility is preferred.

Types of Autopsy

1. Medicolegal Autopsy

This type of autopsy is performed by the doctor on the written instruction from an authorized investigating officer (IO) who is either a police or magistrate of the case falling under the jurisdiction of the area where death has happened. The consent of the relatives of the deceased is neither required nor can they prevent the postmortem examination in such cases. The magistrate or the DCP (Deputy Commissioner of Police) has the authority to waive off the autopsy by a written order in some cases.

Doctor has no such power to waive off postmortem of any case. But in cases where there is high risk of infection (like HIV, rabies, hepatitis, fulminant TB, etc.) from the deceased to the autopsy surgeon and the paramedical staff of the mortuary, the doctor can request the magistrate or DCP in writing for waive off autopsy of the case.

2. Pathological Autopsy

This type of autopsy is performed by a doctor from the department of pathology to know the extent and diagnosis of a disease for which the deceased was being treated while alive. It is also used for academic and research purposes. A written consent of the relatives of the deceased is required in such cases. A relatively newer type of autopsy called Virtopsy is used in a few centers of the world but not in India. It is a non-invasive method of examination of a dead body using imaging techniques like MRI or CT to have a 3D visualization of the tissue and organs of the dead body.

3. Anatomical Autopsy

Anatomical autopsy is done by undergraduate medical students in the department of anatomy to study the various structures and organs of human body.

Guidelines for Medicolegal Autopsy

Doctor should conduct the autopsy after receiving the inquest papers along with the dead body.

1. A single doctor is required to perform an autopsy. However, a board of doctors is constituted by competent authority by order of the magistrate to conduct an autopsy in cases like dowry deaths, custodial deaths, and alleged negligence by the doctor leading to death of the patient.
2. As per National Human Rights Commission all custodial deaths should be videographed and postmortem report should be written in differently designed proforma. The PM report should be handed over to the IO in a sealed envelope after obtaining a receipt.
3. Detailed history of the case should be asked from the IO as well as the inquest papers should be read by the doctor.
4. Autopsy should be done in a fully equipped mortuary of a Government hospital authorized for the purpose. However, in exceptional cases like mass disaster it can be done in open cordoning off and covering the area near the site of disaster.
5. All the three body cavities, viz. skull, chest and abdomen should be opened in every case.
6. No unauthorized person should be allowed inside the autopsy hall.
7. Both the IO and relatives whose names are recorded in the inquest paper should identify the body.
8. It is the duty of the IO to get the body identified.
9. Doctor should recheck the identification.
10. In unknown dead bodies two identification marks should be recorded by the doctor.
11. Autopsy should be carried out preferably in daylight, but doing it in a well-illuminated modern autopsy hall is also acceptable.
12. After completion of the postmortem, the report and the viscera preserved, if any, should be handed over to the IO at the earliest after obtaining a receipt from him.
13. The copy of postmortem report should be maintained in the Department of Forensic Medicine.

Aims and Objectives of Autopsy

1. To find out the cause of death
2. To know the time since death
3. To find the manner of death—suicide, homicide, accidental or natural
4. To find the mode of death—asphyxia, coma or shock

5. To identify the dead body when unknown.
6. To identify the various injuries on the body.
7. To preserve any trace evidence or viscera.
8. In newborn to find out whether dead born, live born, stillborn and age of viability (7th month of IUL) of foetus.
9. To find the sex, age, race and other details of skeletal remains

Procedure for Medicolegal Postmortem

It involves:
1. External examination and
2. Internal examination

External Examination

The following should be examined and noted down.
1. Height, weight and built of the body
2. Match the label of the details on the dead body with those on the inquest paper to avoid doing pm on a wrong dead body.
3. Clothes for any blood, mud, grass, grease, other stains, tear.
4. Identification marks in unknown dead bodies.
5. Natural orifices for any discharge/foreign body.
6. State of rigor mortis—starts usually 2 hours after death. Fully developed in appoximately 12 hours after death, remains in the state of rigor mortis for next 12 hours and then passes off in another 12 hours after death. It can be established by the degree of mobility or stiffening of joints of upper and lower extremity by lifting the middle of upper arm and thigh (Fig. 10.1a). When all the big joints are stiff, it is fully developed. When all the joints are easily flexible, rigor mortis has passed off.
7. Postmortem staining is seen in the dependent parts of the body in the form of patches of about 1–2 cm diameter, bluish-purple or purplish-red color about 30 minutes to 1 hour after death. It is better appreciated in fair complexioned bodies. Postmortem staining gets fixed between 6 and 8 hours after death (Fig. 10.1b and c).

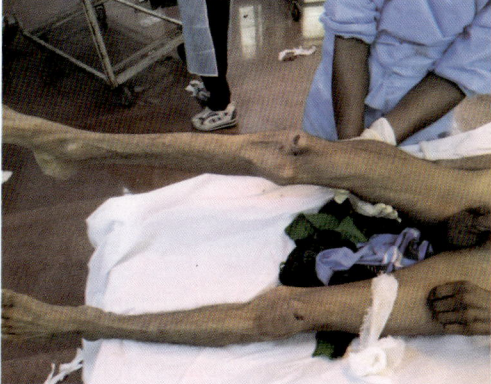 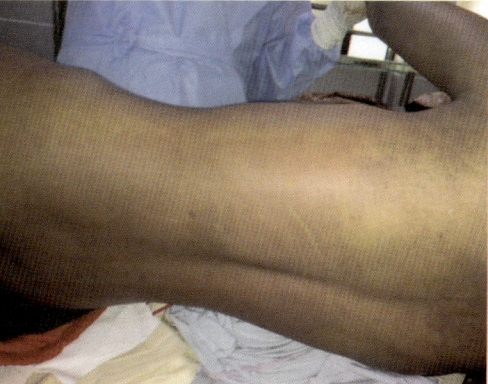

Fig. 10.1a: Demonstration of rigor mortis in the lower limb. No flexion of knee joint on lifting the thigh

Fig. 10.1b: Postmortem staining at the back

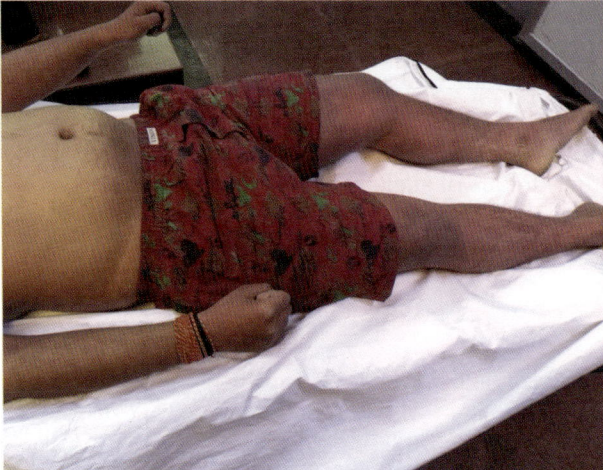

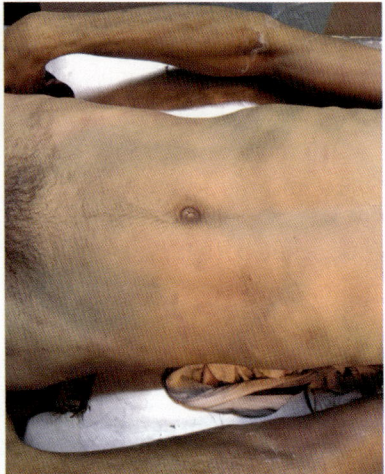

Fig. 10.1c: Postmortem staining in the lower limb in a case of hanging

Fig. 10.2: Early changes of decomposition (bluish discoloration) over abdomen

8. All the external injuries are noted giving each injury a serial number.
9. Decomposition process has started or it is highly decomposed (Fig. 10.2).

After external examination the body should be opened for internal examination by using one of the following types of preliminary skin incisions:

Anterior body wall incisions:

They are of three types:

1. **I-shaped vertical incision:** It starts from symphysis menti with a little curve at the umbilicus down to the symphysis pubis. This incision is most commonly used (Fig. 10.3).
2. **Y-shaped incision:** It starts from xiphisternum to symphysis pubis in midline. The upper end is then extended on the two sides of the chest with an arc at the inframammary region particularly below female breasts and extended upwards up to anterior axillary line on both sides. This incision is usually preferred for cosmetic purposes particularly in females so that no incision mark is visible in the upper part of chest.
3. **Modified Y-shaped incision:** It starts from suprasternal notch to symphysis pubis representing the straight limb of the Y. From the suprasternal notch the incision is extended onto the middle of the clavicle on two sides of the neck terminating at the mastoid processes representing the fork of the Y. This incision is usually preferred in cases of asphyxial deaths due to compression of neck for better visualization of subcutaneous tissue underlying the compressed area.

Posterior Body Wall Incision

It is an **elongated X-shaped incision** on the back of the body with a midline incision over the vertebra starting between the two scapulae and ending between the two posterior superior iliac spines. From the starting points the incision extends to both sides over the scapulae and terminating at the back of both the shoulders forming the upper limbs of the 'X'. The lower two limbs of the 'X' terminating over the right and

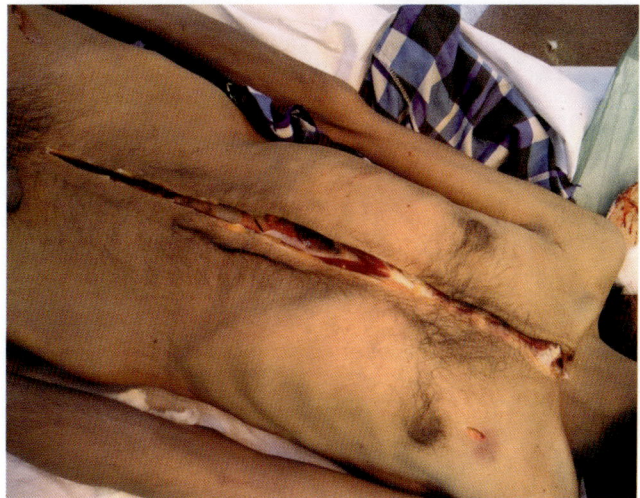

Fig. 10.3: I-shaped midline incision of skin

left gluteal area. This incision is usually used to look for any subcutaneous injury at the back in custody deaths.

Scalp incision: The scalp is incised in the coronal plane from one mastoid to the mastoid on the other side of head. The front portion of the scalp is then pulled up to the upper margin of orbit and back portion of the scalp is pulled up to the occipital protuberance with a gentle sweeping strokes cutting the loose connective tissue of the scalp.

Internal Examination

All the three body cavities must be opened to examine their contents in detail. The body cavities are:

1. Head and neck
2. Chest
3. Abdomen including pelvis.

Different techniques are followed for removal of body organs (evisceration) as follows:

1. **RLK Virchow's technique:** All the organs in this technique are removed one by one. Starting with the cranial cavity, spinal cord followed by thoracic, cervical and abdominal organs. It is the most commonly used method. Individual organs can be studied in details but the anatomical relationships between the organs are not preserved in this method.

2. **C Rokitasky's technique:** It involves a combination of *in-situ* dissection in some part with en-block removal of the other organs. This method is preferred where the autopsy surgeon wants to prevent infection from an organ. But the infected organ cannot be studied in details.

3. **M Letulle's technique:** It involves the en-mass removal of cervical, thoracic, abdominal and pelvic organs and subsequently dissected into organ blocks. It preserves the anatomical relationship between organ and the organ system. It is considered as the best technique.

4. **A Ghon's technique:** In this method the cervicothoracic, abdominal and pelvic organs are removed as three different organ blocks. The organ relationship is well preserved in this technique.

Depending upon the type of case it is the discretion of the autopsy surgeon which of the above techniques he/she chooses. All the organs removed should be weighed and any abnormality found should be recorded. The term 'no abnormality detected' (NAD) should be used when the organ is found normal.

Examination of Head and its Contents

The undersurface of the scalp should be examined for any extravasation of blood (bruise), incised, lacerated, avulsion or firearm wounds. Abrasion of the scalp is not common because of hair, but may be seen in a bald person. The vault of the skull is examined for the following types of fractures:

Fractures of Skull

1. Fissured (linear)—no bony displacement (Fig. 12.1)
2. Depressed (signature)—part of outer table pushed inside the skull caused by blunt force impact (Fig. 12.1).
3. Mosaic (spider web)—radiating linear fracture lines from a depressed fracture.
4. Gutter—caused by tangential trajectory/gliding force, like a bullet.
5. Diastatic (sutural)—fracture at the suture lines.
6. Pond—in a child when the skull is still cartilaginous forming a depression without fracture as in forceps delivery.
7. Ring fracture—fracture encircling the foramen magnum at the base of skull as in fall from height.

Opening the Skull

By using a saw the skull bone is cut in a horizontal plane a little above the glabella in front and occipital protuberance at the back. Both the cut edges are continued and meet at an angle of 120° at the mastoid process. The part of the skull thus removed is called skull cap. The skull cap is examined for any fractures.

Removal and Examination of Brain

After removing the skull cap the dura mater covering the brain becomes visible (Fig. 12.2).
1. The surface of the dura is examined for any extradural/epidural hemorrhage (Fig. 12.8) (above the dura), edema, yellowish/greenish color indicating pus formation or decomposition in the brain. When edematous the dura will be full and tense.
2. The superior sagittal sinus is incised with a scalpel and examined for any thrombus.
3. The dura mater is cut with a pair of scissors on either side of midline of brain from frontal to occipital lobe and also along the coronal plane side to side. The four flaps of dura are then examined for any subdural hemorrhage (which can be easily washed away with water, Fig. 12.4) or subarachnoid hemorrhage (which cannot be washed away with water, Figs 12.5, 12.17a and b).

4. The falx cerebri is then freed from the cribriform plate and pulled backwards. The frontal lobes of the brain are now lifted by inserting four fingers of one hand under it and with the other hand the optic chiasma and other cranial nerves are cut as far away from the base of the brain as possible.

5. The tentorium cerebri is cut on both sides and cervical cord below the medulla is cut through the foramen magnum. The brain is then gently removed by using both the hands by cutting the remaining dura attached to the base of the skull. One hand is used as a support to hold the brainstem and cerebellum and other hand to support the frontal and parietal lobes to deliver the brain out of the skull cavity. The brain is then weighed.

   Normal weight of brain in adults is between 1200 and 1400 gm. In newborn it is between 350 and 400 gm.

6. Examine the base of the skull for ring fracture around foramen magnum. Fractures in anterior, middle and posterior cranial fossa or any transverse fracture (Fig. 8.3).

7. The brain is preferably fixed in freshly prepared 10% formalin solution for study of anatomical structures.

8. The circle of Willis at the base of the fixed brain, other cerebral vessels are examined for any embolism, thrombus or aneurysm.

9. The cerebral hemisphere is then sliced using brain knife in the coronal plane with a thickness of about 1 cm from the frontal to the occipital lobe (Fig. 12.16). The white matter is examined for any petechial hemorrhage as often seen in fat embolism. When **edematous the weight of the brain is more than 1450 gm** (Figs 12.6, 12.11), midline shift, sulci will be shallow and narrow, gyri flattened and uncal herniation. Cut section of the brain will show the grey matter as a thin line being pushed towards the periphery by the white matter (Figs 12.6, 12.11 and 12.16).

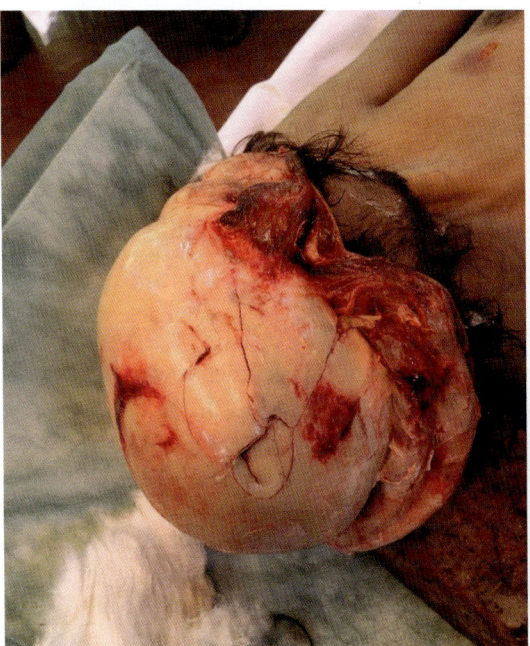

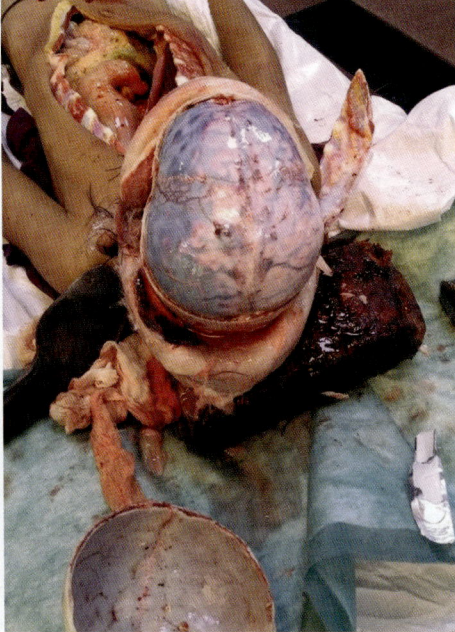

Fig. 12.1: Skull showing fissured and depressed fracture   **Fig. 12.2:** Skull cap removed. Dura mater with bluish tint covering the brain

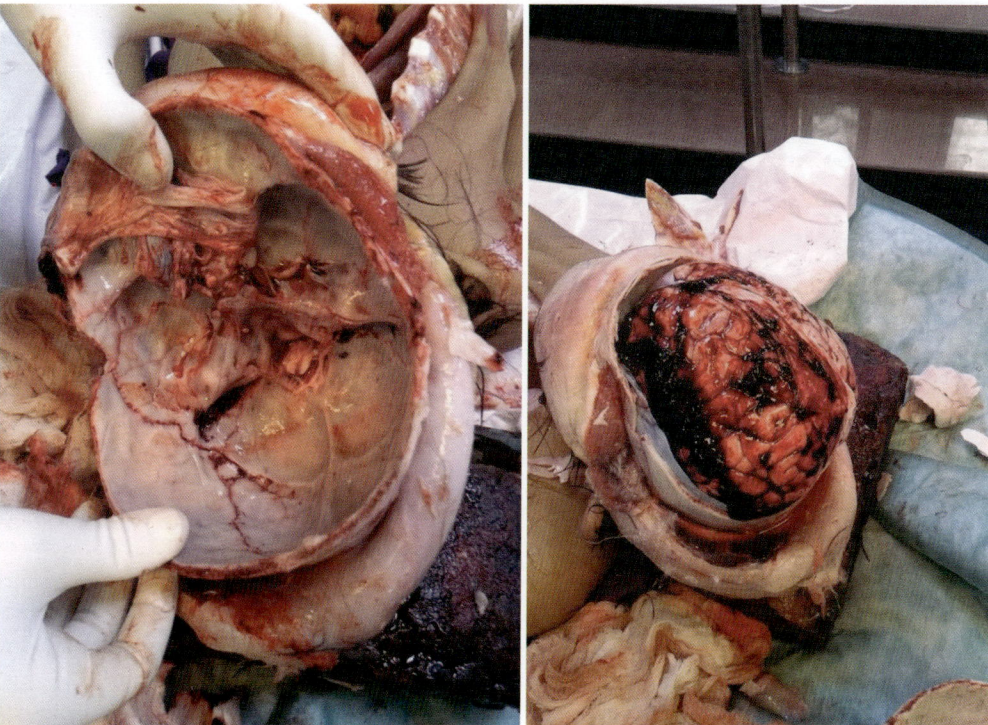

Fig. 12.3: Fracture base of skull   **Fig. 12.4:** Brain showing subdural hemorrhage

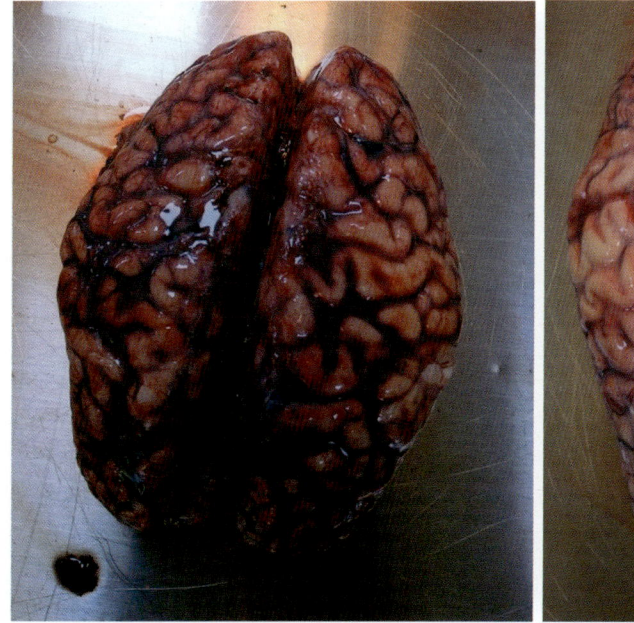

Fig. 12.5: Brain showing subarachnoid hemorrhage

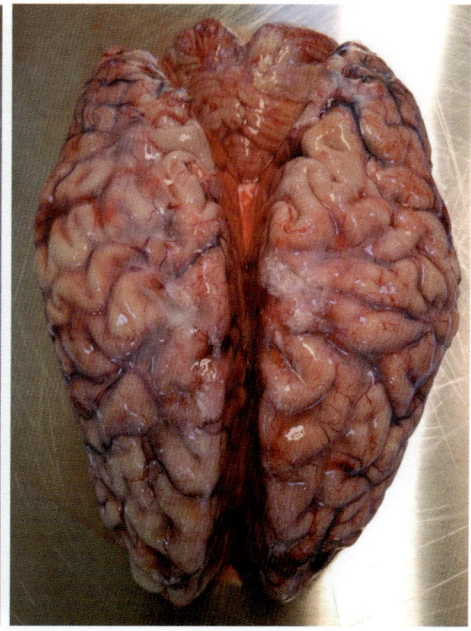

Fig. 12.6: Edematous brain

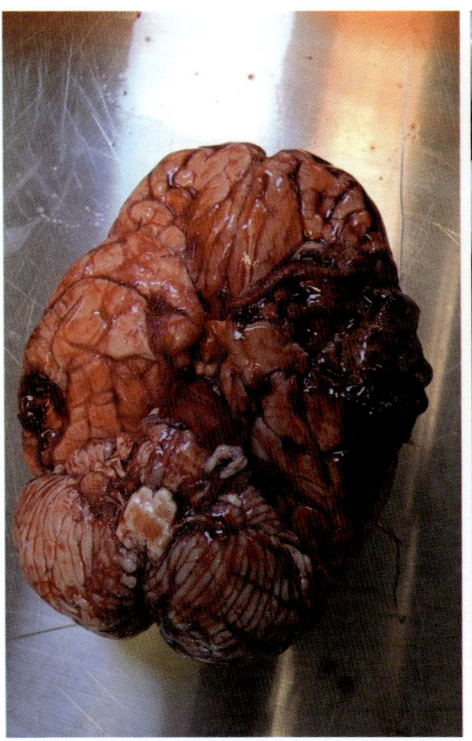

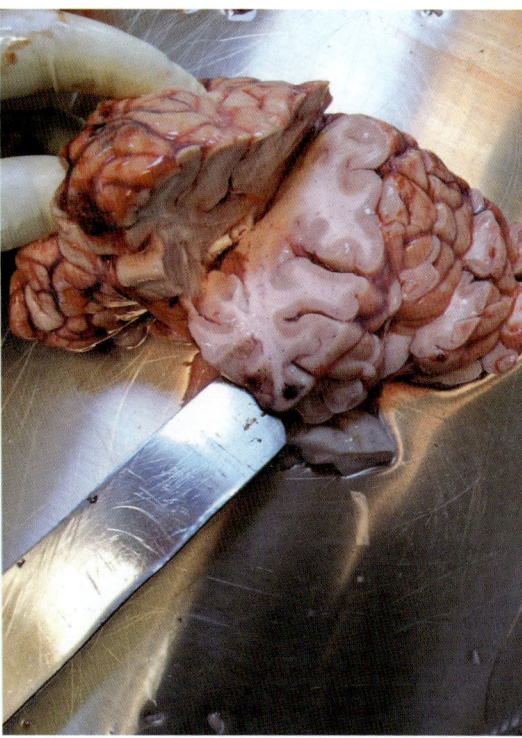

Fig. 12.7: Inferior surface of brain with extradural hemorrhage

Fig. 12.8: Brain showing intracerebral hemorrhage

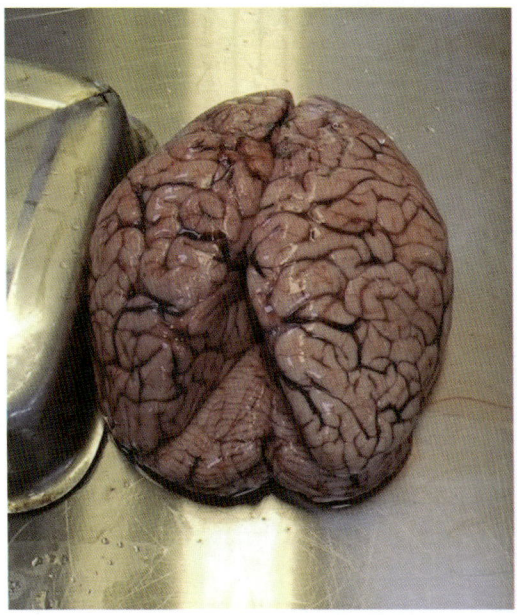

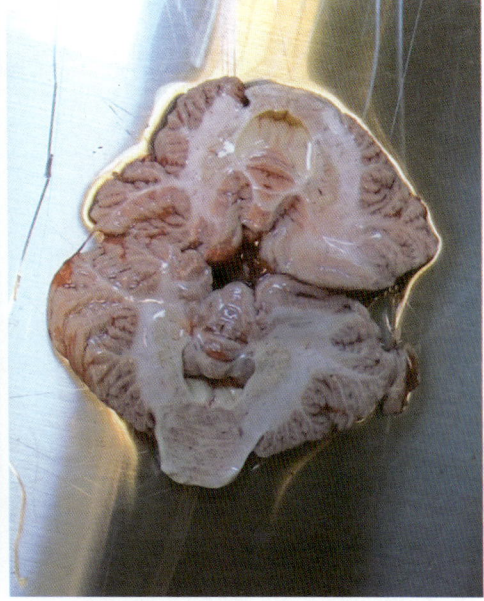

Fig. 12.9: Normal brain

Fig. 12.10: Cut section of normal cerebellum

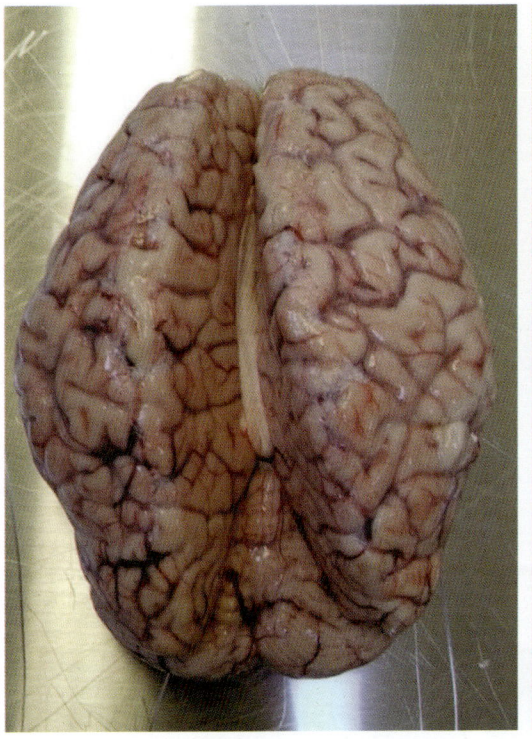

Fig. 12.11: Edematous brain

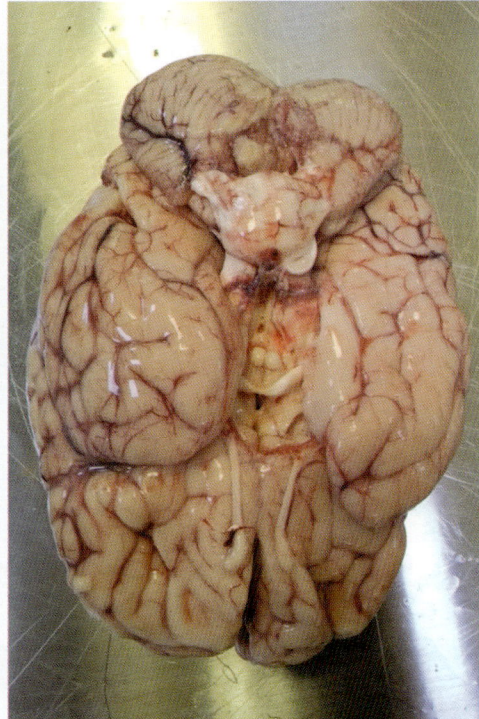

Fig. 12.12: Inferior surface of brain

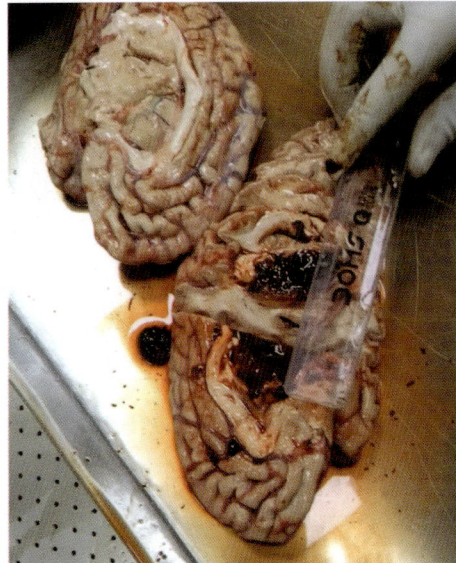

Fig. 12.13: Hemorrhage in fourth ventricle of brain

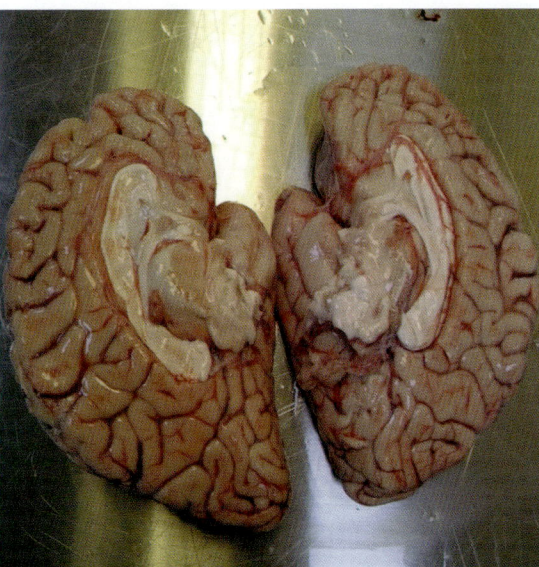

Fig. 12.14: Vertical cut section of brain showing corpus callosum

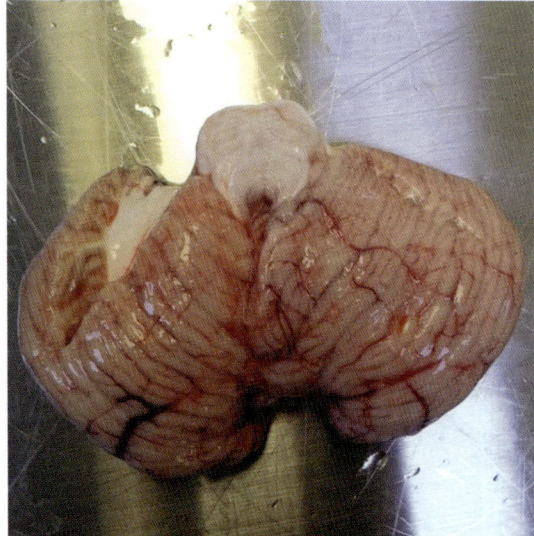

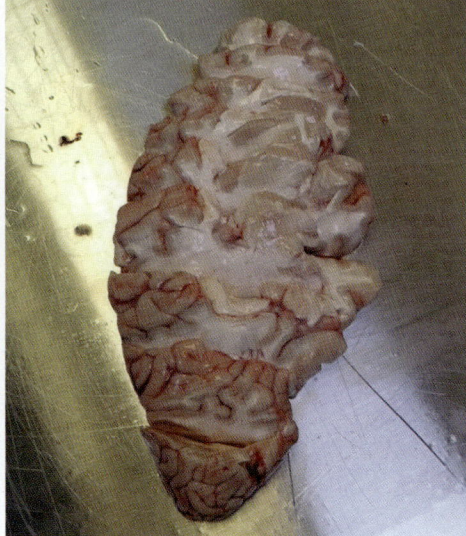

Fig. 12.15: Cerebellum showing cut section of midbrain

Fig. 12.16: Vertical section of half of cerebral hemisphere showing white and gray matter

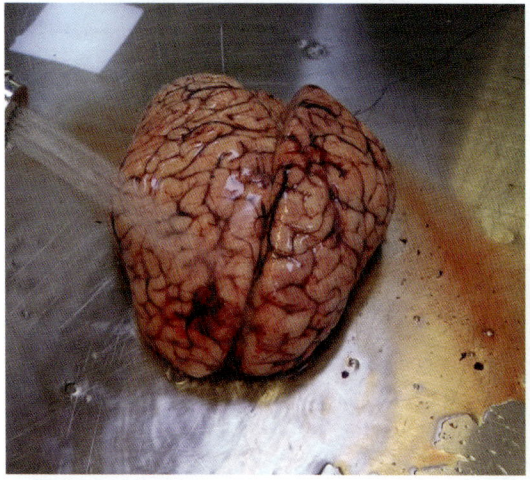

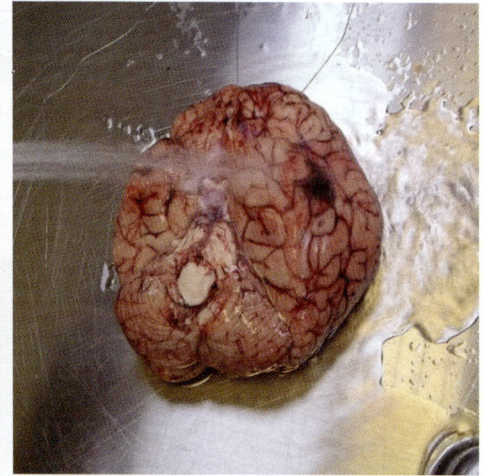

Fig. 12.17a: Subarachnoid hemorrhage

Fig. 12.17b: Subarachnoid hemorrhage in brain

Causes of cerebral edema: Brain trauma, tumors, focal inflammation and infection, cerebral ischemia, stroke by blood clot, encephalopathy, high altitude, hypoxia, hydrocephalus (obstructive type), glioma, meningitis, hyponatremia, CO poisoning, viral infection.

10. The cerebrum can also be examined by dissecting in the sagittal plane (Fig. 12.14). It is useful for the examination of the 3rd and 4th ventricle (Fig. 12.13). Using a scalpel it is cut through the corpus callosus starting at the genu and then extending the cut upwards through the midline of the brainstem and bisecting the basilar artery on the ventral surface of the pons.

11. The cerebellum and brainstem are separated from the cerebrum by cutting the cerebral peduncles (Fig. 12.10).

12. The cerebellum is dissected in the horizontal plane and brainstem perpendicular to its axis (Fig. 12.15).
13. When some infection and cerebral poisoning is suspected, the brain should be dissected in the sagittal plane in the midline exposing the corpus callosum and fornices. When fresh for microbiological and chemical examination, it is then reflected backwards to examine the thalamus and caudate nucleus (Fig. 12.8).
14. Any intracerebral hemorrhage should be looked for by exposing each slice of brain on the right of the autopsy surgeon.
15. The fourth ventricle is exposed by cutting along the vermis in midline using a scalpel.
16. The internal, external capsule and basal ganglia are now examined.
17. The pons, medulla and part of cervical cord are examined by making horizontal section.

Any asymmetry or brain shift indicates a large SOL such as abscesses, hemorrhage recent infarct and primary or metastatic tumors. Cystic spaces or old infarct do not produce any brain shift in spite of being large size.

Removal of Pituitary Gland

The pituitary fossa which lies between the sphenoid bones called sella turcica in the base of the skull is inspected. It remains covered by diaphragma sella. The posterior wall of the sphenoid bone is broken using a clamp or a pair of forceps. A blunt instrument or a scalpel is inserted into the fossa as low as possible from the side. The pituitary gland is now elevated and delivered superiorly in an intact form without being crushed.

Pituitary gland is examined for size, weight and any atrophy or hyperplasia.

Normal size of pituitary: –2 × 1.5 × 0.5 cm, weight—500–600 gm.

Removal of Spinal Cord

It can be removed both by anterior and posterior approach. Posterior approach is preferred as it is easy and quicker. It should be performed before opening the anterior of the body to avoid spillage of tissues and organs from anterior body cavities while turning the body. A midline incision is made while the body is in prone position starting from occiput to the coccyx. Vertebral column is then exposed by removing the soft tissue. The exposed laminae of the vertebral bodies are then cut with a saw directed forwards and slightly inwards placed at a distance of 2 cm away from midline on either side. As soon as the saw gives in it should be withdrawn to be exposed which ensures the saw is in correct plane and position. Horizontal cuts should be made in upper cervical region and at the sacral region below. The vertebral column can now be lifted free after chipping away the bone with forceps which will expose the cord alongwith dura sufficiently to allow its removal. The lumbar region should be gently gripped with artery forceps and the cord distal to the cauda equina transected using a scalpel. After removal from the vertebral canal the cord is fixed in formalin for four weeks. The dura covering the cord should be opened anteriorly using a small pair of scissors and the cord examined externally. The blocks of the cord are then sliced at 5 mm interval in between the nerve roots. It is then sent for histopathological examination.

Length of spinal cord—45 cm, weight—26–27 gm.

Examination of Neck

Neck circumference should be measured lifting the hair particularly in females from the back.

Externally the neck should be examined for:
a. Ligature material *in situ* if present.
b. Ligature mark—LxBxD position, above/below thyroid cartilage, complete/incomplete, color, parchmentization.
c. Finger nail marks—crescentic abrasions seen in throttling (manual strangulation)
   Internal examination of neck is done by keeping a 10–15 cm high block placed under shoulder of the cadaver which allows complete extension of neck. It should be done gently to avoid subluxation of C6–C7 vertebrae due to tearing of intervertebral disc known as **undertaker's fracture**. This is a postmortem injury.
   Neck structures are freed by passing a knife under the skin from the midline incision until it enters the floor of mouth. The knife is then run around inside of the mandible to free the tongue. The tissues at the back and sides of the pharynx are divided and

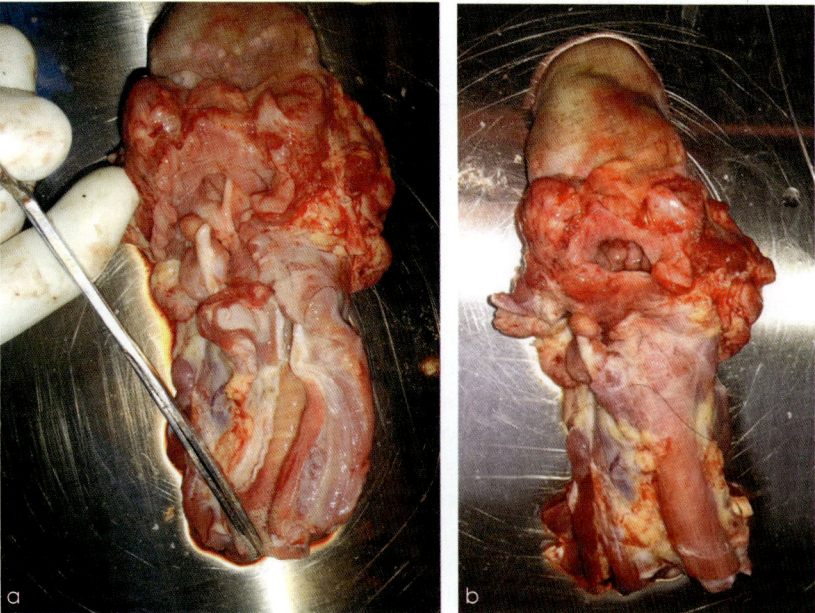

Fig. 13.1: (a) Trachea cut open showing normal mucosa with tracheal ring; (b) soft tissues of the neck along with the tongue

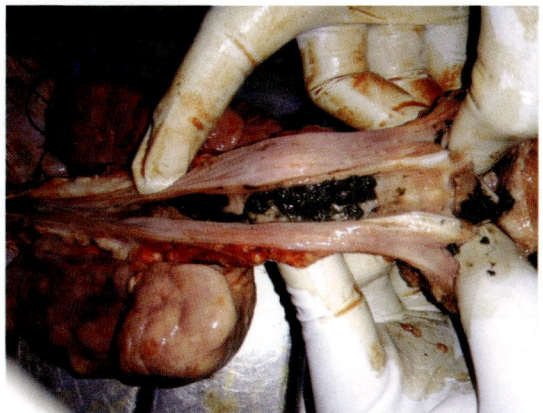

Fig. 13.2: Shoot particles in trachea in antemortem burn

tonsillar area cut through. Fingers are then passed up behind the symphysis menti to grasp the tongue, which is then drawn down by dividing the tissues behind the larynx to release the neck structures. The pharynx and glottis are looked for any bleeding, obstruction and edema (Fig. 13.1a and 13.1b). The platysma muscles are examined for any bruising. External jugular vein is examined and the underlying muscles are reflected in layers. First the sternal head of sternocleidomastoid muscles are divided from the manubrium. The carotid sheet, carotid artery, internal jugular vein and vagus nerve are exposed after the omohyoid muscle is reflected and examined for any injury or hemorrhage. The hyoid bone (after 40 years of age) should be examined for any fracture (demonstrated by mobility of the fracture ends) after detaching it from various muscles attached to it. Fracture is commonly seen in manual and sometimes in ligature strangulation. Trachea should be cut vertically with a pair of scissors and the mucosa is examined for congestion, tracheal ring or any shoot particles (Figs 13.1a and 13.2). The cut is then extended up to the bronchioles from the bifurcation of right and left bronchus.

Examination of Chest Cavity and its Contents—Heart and Lungs

1. From the midline incision the skin over the chest is retracted laterally on both sides exposing the rib cage up to anterior axillary line and at the upper end exposing the clavicle.
2. The sternoclavicular joint is identified by gentle manipulation of the clavicle which is disarticulated by a scalpel. The costochondral junction of the 1st rib is cut using a rib cutter.
3. Along the line of the 1st rib the costochondral junction of the rest of the ribs are cut using a rib shear just medial to the cartilage to avoid exposing sharp edges of the rib bones.
4. The sternal plate/flap is then removed by cutting from below upwards taking care not to damage the mediastinal soft tissues (Fig. 14.1). The undersurface of skin of the chest is looked for any extravasation of blood. The ribs and sternum are examined. for any fracture. The mediastinum is examined for any blood and injuries. **Pneumothorax** can be demonstrated by using a no. 20 needle attached to a 50 ml syringe without the piston containing water. The needle of the above syringe is then inserted into an intercostal space. If air is present in the pleural cavity, air bubble will be seen in the water of the syringe.
5. The chest cavity after removal of sternal flap is retracted and presence of any liquid and clotted blood is noted. Quantity of blood is measured. The blood, if any, is then

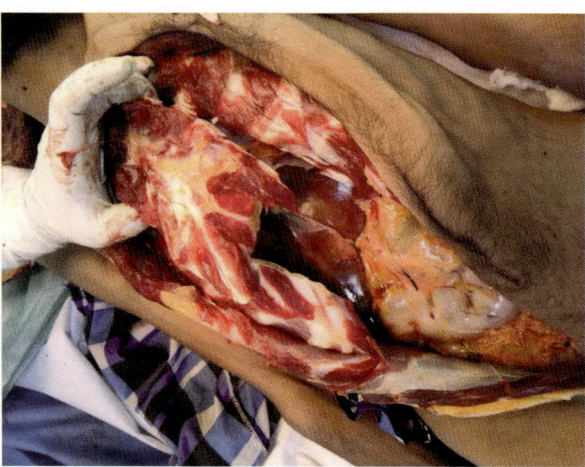

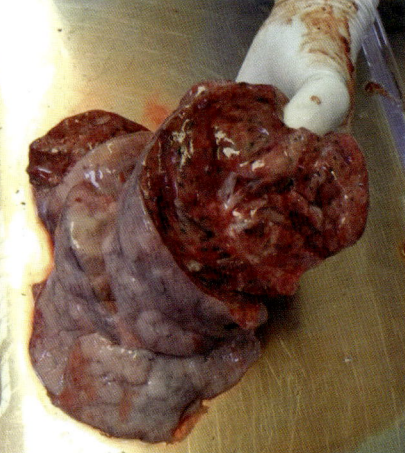

Fig. 14.1: Removal of sternal flap by cutting the costo-chondral junction on both sides. Underlying liver and intestines are visible in the abdominal cavity

Fig. 14.2: Cut section of lungs showing congested parenchyma with pus pockets

removed from the chest cavity to get a clear picture of its contents. The pericardial surface of heart and pleural surface of both the lungs are examined for collection of any fluid or blood. All pleural attachments should be removed by blunt dissection. If parietal pleura are firmly attached to the lungs it has to be stripped with the lungs. A firmly adherent fibrous band of parietal pleura indicates old tubercular infection, chronic lung disease, a pleural or underlying lung tumor or metastasis.

6. The lungs are removed by freeing it from all the pleural attachments, lifted forward out of the pleural cavity and the root held with the noncutting hand while the dominant hand is used to cut through the hilar tissue to detach lung through primary bronchus, vessels and pleura.

Normal consistency of the lungs is described as sponge like.

Normal weight of lungs—Right: 350–550 gm, Left: 325–425 gm

Lungs weighing more than 1 kg is seen

a. Severe cardiac failure

b. Severe pneumonia (hepatization or liver-like consistency of the lungs)

c. Diffuse alveolar damage (drowning)

Examination of Lungs

The lung surface is looked for congestion, petechial hemorrhage, particularly in the interlobar surface (asphyxia or poisoning deaths) and emphysematous bullae. Green or yellowish color indicates purulent material.

The primary bronchial mucosa is examined for any congestion, lumen for shoot particles mixed with mucus (antemortem burns death, *see* Fig. 13.2), foreign body (choking deaths) or dirty liquid (drowning deaths). The bronchus from its bifurcation is cut by a pair of scissors from medial to lateral up to the bronchioles in the lung parenchyma of all the lobes to look for changes as described for bronchus.

Old tubercular cavities and fungal balls can also be demonstrated by dissecting the airways as described.

Slicing of the lungs is done by making horizontal dissection through each lobe using a brain knife. Lung parenchyma of each slice is examined for oozing of frothy fluid **(edema)**, pockets of pus **(septicemia)**, bloody froth **(asphyxia)**, and **tubercles** (Fig. 14.2). When no obvious pathology is found, the slices should be sent for histological examination to rule out asbestosis, pneumoconiosis. For demonstration of presence of chronic obstructive pulmonary disease (COPD), the slices are fixed and their appearance is examined by using a hand lens. Air spaces measuring more than 1 mm indicate emphysema.

Pulmonary edema is fluid collection in the tissues and alveoli of lungs.

Causes of Pulmonary Edema

Cardiogenic

- LVF due to myocardial damage, e.g. MI
- Cardiomyopathy
- Mitral stenosis
- Aortic regurgitation
- Hypertension

Noncardiogenic

- Blunt trauma to chest wall
- Head injury (intracranial hemorrhage, severe seizures)
- Pneumonia/lung infection
- Pulmonary embolism
- Pneumothorax
- Rapid drainage of large pulmonary effusion
- Drowning
- High altitude
- Kidney disease
- Septicemia
- Inhalation of toxins such as ammonia, parathion, chloride, cocaine, methadone, heroin
- Aspirin
- Acute respiratory distress syndrome (ARDS)
- Dengue and Hantavirus infection.
- Eclampsia in pregnancy.
- Adverse reaction to drugs

Examination of Pulmonary Blood Vessels

The horizontal and oblique fissures of lungs are identified and the hilar segment of each pulmonary artery is identified deep within the soft tissue of the fissure. The lumen of the vessels is cut by scissor in the peripheral direction like used for opening the airways. Any emboli or atheroma present is looked for. Antemortem embolus is seen as a coiled mass, when straightened it resembles the cast of the vessel of origin of thrombus as in deep vein thrombosis. Antemortem thrombus will be firmly adherent to the endothelial lining of the blood vessel. It is made up of alternating layers of platelet and fibrin. Postmortem thrombus is loosely adherent, red in color and friable.

Removal of Heart from Chest Cavity

The apex of the heart is held with one hand, lifted upwards and separated from the thoracic organs. The other hand is used for cutting the inferior and superior vena cava, pulmonary blood vessels and ascending aorta as far distal from the base of the heart as possible. It is then taken out of the chest cavity and placed on a tray in the anatomical position. Its weight, size and shape are noted. The weight should be taken after all the blood clots in the chambers of the heart has been removed to avoid any elevated weight.

Normal weight of the heart is: 250 to 300 gm.

Normal size of heart is: Length—11.5–12.5 cm (from apex to base)

Breadth: 9–10 cm (at AV groove)

External Examination of Heart

The epicardial surface should be examined for evidence of pericarditis, focal hyperemia, rupture and flaccidity, which may indicate underlying infarct. Presence of small white patches over the right ventricle anteriorly indicates previous trauma or subclinical pericarditis. The color of the surface may be greenish yellow indicating either a part of generalized or local infective process. Petechial hemorrhage indicates asphyxia/ septicemia.

Normal pericardial fluid is straw colored and 5–15 ml in volume. In pericardial effusion/tamponade it may increase to 1 liter when there is slow collection of fluid in the pericardial sac. If collection is fast, even 200 ml can be fatal.

Examination of coronary arteries: The coronary arteries should be examined before the chambers of the heart because of their external disposition on the surface.

Anatomy of Coronary Arteries

The origin of the left main coronary artery is identified externally between the aorta and left atria. It soon divides into left circumflex and left anterior descending artery. The left circumflex artery runs in the groove between left atrium and left ventricle anteriorly and becomes difficult to identify posteriorly. The left anterior descending artery runs in the septal groove between the left and right ventricles and becoming unidentifiable near the apex of heart. The right coronary artery is the most difficult to find, as it is often embedded within a large amount of epicardial fat. It emerges between the right atrium and pulmonary trunk, runs posteriorly in the atrioventricular groove between right atrium and ventricle and then turns inferiorly to run in the posterior septal groove, where it goes to the apex of the heart and supplies blood to the posterior septal wall.

Dissection of Coronary Arteries

The right and left coronary ostia are first identified by inspecting the aortic sinuses from above (Figs 14.4, 14.8 and 14.9). A finger is passed through the cut end of aorta and ostia are palpated for presence of any thrombus or calcification. The coronary arteries are cut with a scalpel in cross-sections starting 1 cm away from the origin of left coronary artery at an interval of 3–5 mm to evaluate atherosclerotic narrowing of the lumen (Fig. 14.3).

An occlusion less than 50% is considered mild, between 50% and 75% moderate and more than 75% is severe. A four-point grading system is also applied by 25% increment in narrowing. A 75% occlusion is grade-4 which is considered severe and a 90% occlusion is considered critical. When heavily calcified, the vessels need to be transected using a sharp pair of artery scissors (Figs 14.3 and 14.6).

Dissection of Heart

The heart is usually opened along the flow of blood as follows:

1. A transverse incomplete slice is made 3 cm away from the apex of heart on the ventricle. The inside of both the ventricular chambers are visible from the cut end.
2. The right atrium is opened anteriorly by cutting from the free end of the inferior vena cava to the tip of atrial appendage.
3. The right ventricle is then cut along the free lateral border through the tricuspid ring continuing up to the apex.
4. The pulmonary outflow tract is then opened by a cut in the anterior wall of right ventricle starting at the apex continuing up to the pulmonary conus, valve and artery.

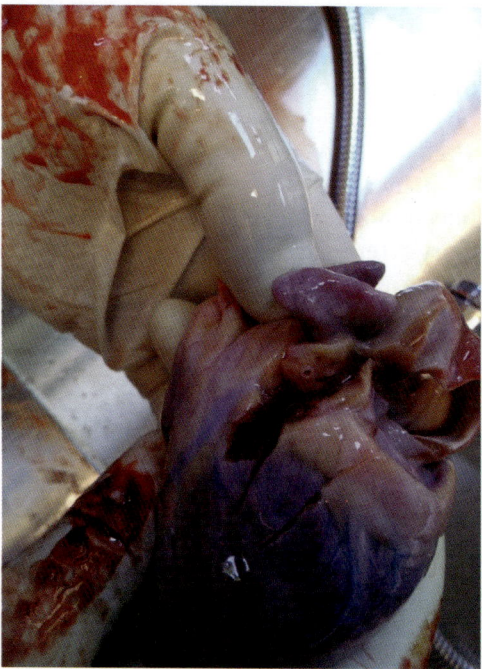

Fig. 14.3: Heart showing patent coronary artery (circumflex)

5. The left atrium is opened by making a hole in the atrial appendage and then extending it to a cut parallel with and above the AV groove.
6. The left ventricle is opened by cutting along the free lateral border through the mitral valve ring and continuing to the apex. The anterior mitral valve cusps are left intact.
7. The outflow tract is now opened by cutting from the apex along the anterior wall of the left ventricle as close to the septal wall as possible and then through the aortic valve up to the open end of aorta.

Internal Examination of the Heart

1. The endocardium should be examined for any fibrosis due to previous pathology like MI or endocarditis.
2. Atrial appendages should be examined for the presence of any thrombus the most common site.
3. The valves including number of cusps, adhesions between cusps, vegetation, fibrosis or calcifications should be looked for (Figs 14.5–14.7).

   Normal circumference of valves
   a. Mitral—10 cm (admits 2 fingers)
   b. Tricuspid—12 cm (admits 3 fingers)
   c. Aortic—7.5 cm (mean)
   d. Pulmonary—8.5 cm (mean)
   Increase in valve circumference suggests—regurgitation/incompetence
   Decrease in valve circumference suggests—stenosis

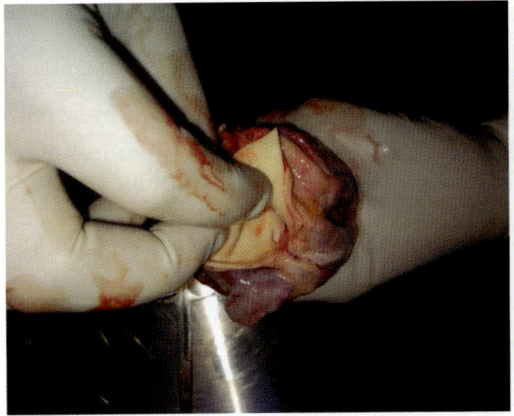

Fig. 14.4: Right coronary ostia at the base of aorta

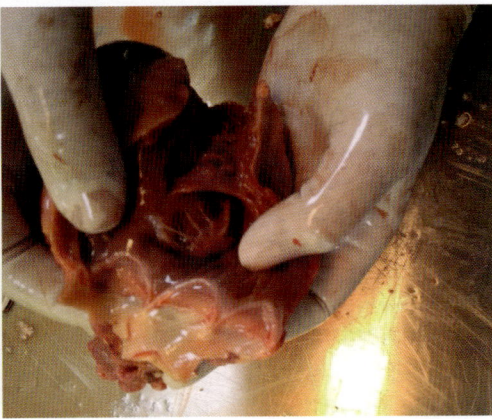

Fig. 14.5: Pulmonary valve with 3 cusps

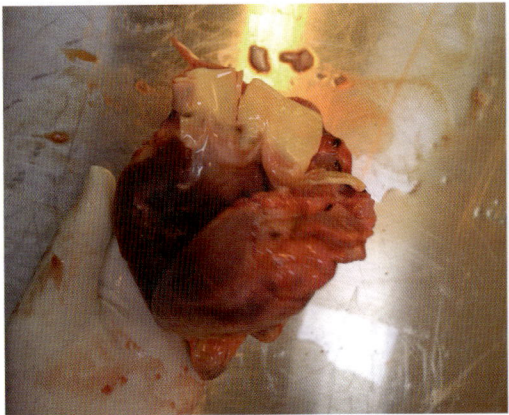

Fig. 14.6: Cusps of aortic valve

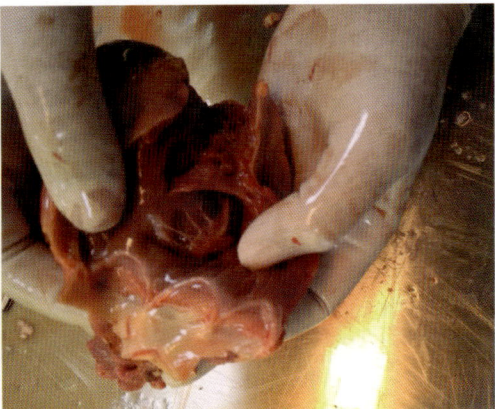

Fig. 14.7: Cusps of pulmonary valve

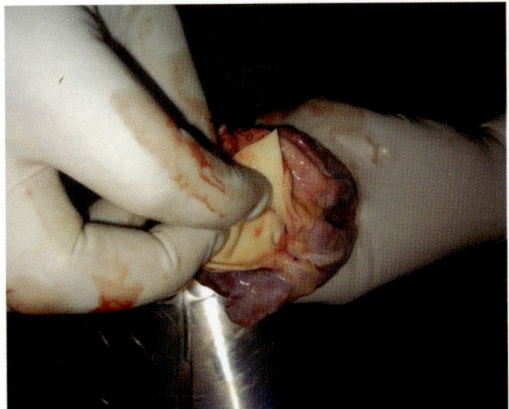

Fig. 14.8: Left coronary ostia at the base of aorta

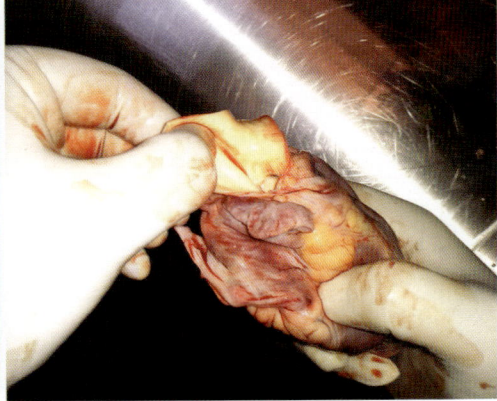

Fig. 14.9: Right coronary ostia at the base of aorta

4. Myocardium should be examined for areas of fibrosis (due to old infarct) or recent infarct. An infarct less than 12 hours cannot be grossly identified. However, a dye (TTC: Triphenyltetrazolium chloride) with dubious validity has been used in such cases. An infarct between 12 and 24 hours is identifiable as a softened area with dusky, hemorrhagic discoloration. Between 1 and 4 days the infarct has a mottled yellow/red pattern. On cut section the infarcted area has a granular and pale appearance with loss of normal luster.

5. Any ventricular hypertrophy should be assessed by measuring the thickness of the ventricular wall.

Normal ventricular and atrial thickness
a. Left ventricle—1.5 cm
b. Right ventricle—0.5 cm
c. Atrial muscle—0.3 cm

Ventricular hypertrophy is seen in
a. Coronary ischemia
b. Hypertension
c. Valvular disease
d. COPD

CHAPTER

15

Examination of Abdominal Cavity and its Contents

The abdominal cavity is opened by a midline incision of the rectus abdominis muscle. Next index and middle finger of the non-cutting hand is introduced into the peritoneal cavity after making a nick in the peritoneum. The abdominal wall is then lifted and the cut is extended upwards up to xiphisternum and downwards up to pubic symphysis. The abdominal cavity is now clearly visible.

The cavity is looked for the presence of:

a. Straw colored translucent fluid due to peritonitis usually caused by perforation of stomach or intestines

b. Pus-yellowish/greenish colored—caused by bacterial or fungal infection

c. Blood—liquid/clotted/extravasation caused by rupture of blood vessels due to trauma. Quantity of above fluid should be measured.

d. Adhesions of intestinal loops/viscera indicates chronic infective process.

e. Obstruction or gangrene of intestines.

f. Foreign body like bullet, pellet, broken knife blade, torn suture material in post-operative cases and food material in gastric perforation.

Removal of Liver

It is done by passing the left hand between the right lobe of the liver and the diaphragm and the liver is pushed forward out of the right hypochondrium. It is now grasped by placing the thumb under the lower anterior border and the remaining fingers are inserted into the long incision for grip. The liver is now lifted and cut through its various ligamentous attachments and the soft tissues between liver and right kidney. The liver can now be removed from the abdominal cavity (Figs 15.1–15.3). It is then weighed and abnormalities like injuries, diseases including cirrhosis, metastatic tumors with hepatomegaly, inflammatory conditions, fatty liver, congenital anomalies, cysts and hemangiomas are looked for.

Normal weight of the liver is 1200 to 1400 gm in an adult.

Dissection of liver—a series of parallel vertical slices are made approximately 2 cm apart from one to the other end of the liver. Sweeping slices are made by a large bladed knife with an uninterrupted pulling motion through the full thickness of parenchyma. If any abnormality is detected, a block of liver is kept for histopathological examination (Fig.15.4). In cases of suspected poisoning, liver tissue or sometimes the whole liver is preserved for toxicological analysis. Gall bladder is examined on the under surface of liver. Ampulla of Vater which opens in the duodenum is examined by pressing the gall bladder. Bile oozes out if bile duct is patent, no oozing if bile duct is blocked by a calculus. Bile duct is opened using a small pair of scissors.

73

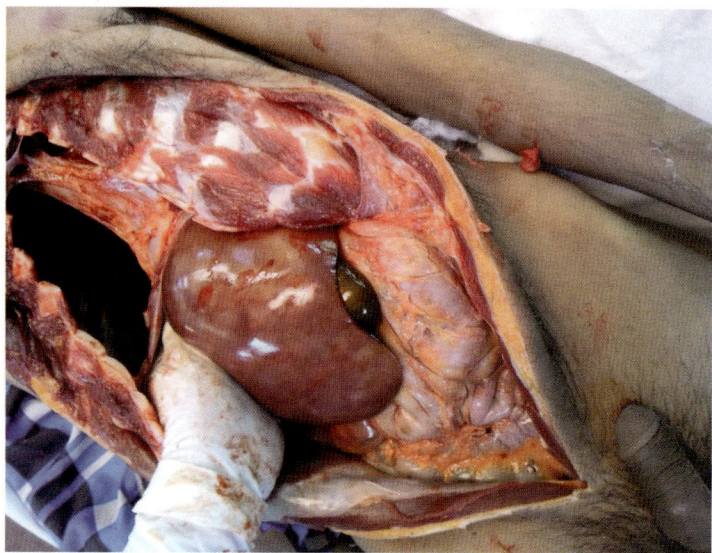

Fig. 15.1: Liver with gall bladder and intestines in abdominal cavity

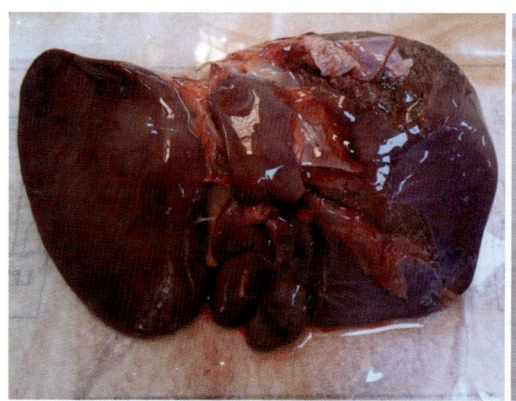

Fig. 15.2: Inferior surface of normal liver

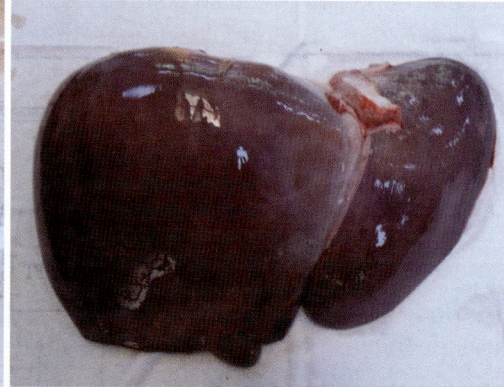

Fig. 15.3: Normal liver

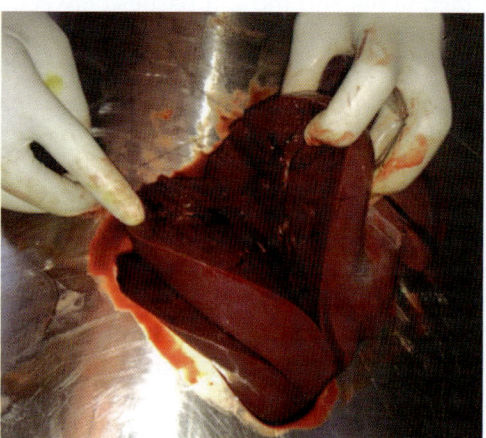

Fig. 15.4: Cut section of liver

Examination of Pancreas

It is a retroperitoneal organ. It lies horizontally below the stomach along the 'C' loop of the duodenum from head to tail. It can be recognized by its pale yellowish glandular appearance.

Normal weight of pancreas is about 100 gm.

The pancreas is identified by lifting the anterior wall of the stomach and palpating the posterior soft tissues. The soft tissues around the pancreas are dissected away and the organ removed. Pancreas is opened by cutting along the main pancreatic duct with a small pair of scissors from ampulla towards the tail. It is cut by making vertical and parallel slices from one to the other end. Any pancreatic mass, hemorrhage, inflammatory changes should be looked and sent for histopathological examination. The pancreas can be lacerated in abdominal injuries releasing the autolytic enzyme that can cause autodigestion of part of pancreas and surrounding tissues. Inflammatory disease of pancreas may be associated with fat necrosis which can be demonstrated by bathing the tissue in concentrated copper acetate solution and incubating it for 24 to 48 hours. The tissue will turn blue-green in color when there is fat necrosis.

Removal of Spleen

Spleen is present in the left hypochondrium just below the undersurface of diaphragm between the 9th and the 11th ribs. It can be easily removed by putting the fingers of right hand between the upper surface of spleen and gently pulling it forwards detaching its attachments.

Normal weight of spleen is 100 to 200 gm.

Examination of Spleen

It should be examined for enlargement (splenomegaly), hemorrhage due to trauma or spontaneous. Spleen is the reservoir of more than half of body's monocytes which act as macrophages and helps in healing of infections caused by micro-organisms. A block of spleen is preserved in cases of death due to septicemia during autopsy for histopathological examination of the macrophages and micro-organisms. Spleen is then sliced using brain knife to examine its parenchyma for any congestion or pus pockets (Fig. 15.7).

Splenomegaly may be due to:
1. Malaria
2. CML
3. Hemolytic anemia
4. Hodgkin's disease
5. CLL
6. Infectious mononucleosis

Examination of Mesentery

It is normally a transparent sheet of tissue with mesenteric blood vessels covering the intestines. The blood vessels may get ruptured in heavy blunt trauma to the abdomen wherein the intestines are also involved. In cases of septicemia its color becomes yellowish green and no more look transparent. Mesenteric lymphadenopathy may be seen in abdominal tuberculosis.

Examination of Stomach

The stomach should be examined externally for any perforation, oozing out of gastric contents, hemorrhagic patches.

Removal and Examination of Stomach and its Contents

Both the cardiac end (esophageal end) and the pyloric end (duodenal end) are tied with a ligature so that the stomach contents do not spill over after its removal. It is cut proximal to the cardiac and distal to the pyloric ends and the stomach is removed from the abdominal cavity and placed on clean tray (Fig. 15.5a). The stomach is then cut along the greater curvature and its contents examined after it is emptied in the clean tray (Fig. 15.5b). Liquids from esophagus generally pass along the lesser curvature of the stomach straightaway into the duodenum and then to intestines. Therefore, poisoning by any corrosive liquid will cause ulceration along the lesser curvature of stomach. For this reason the stomach must be opened along the greater curvature so as to visualize the ulceration along the lesser curvature. The mucosal wall should be examined for hemorrhagic patch, congestion, ulceration, stain or perforation which are usually seen in cases of poisoning, asphyxial deaths, stab or firearm injuries. The state of digestion of food material in the stomach should be noted which help in assessing the time since death. Usually food is completely digested in the stomach by 4 to 6 hours depending on the type of food.

Examination of Intestines

The external surface should be examined from the jejunum to rectum after isolating the intestines with or without mesentery for any contusion, perforation and obstruction. The internal examination is done by opening the intestines along the antimesenteric border using a bowel scissors having a hooked end to stop slipping of the bowel during opening. It can be opened either from the duodenal or rectal end. Any local mass or tumor, diverticula should be looked for. The tumor tissues should be sent for histopathological examination. Surgical sutures in postoperative cases and whether they are intact, loose or torn should be noted. Adhesions of the intestinal loops with each other and mesentery indicate some abdominal infection like tuberculosis and

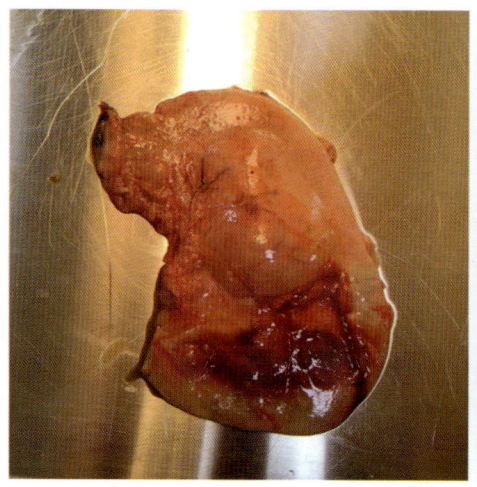

Fig. 15.5a: Intact stomach

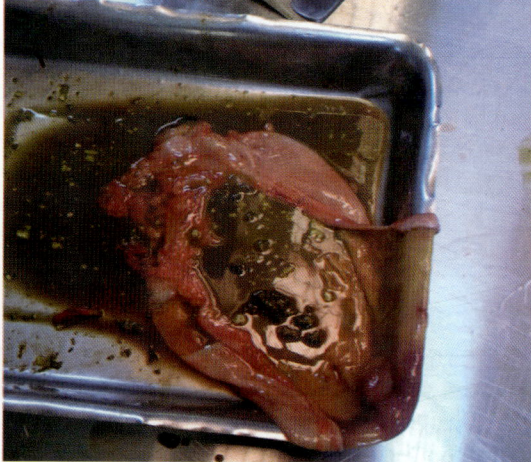

Fig. 15.5b: Stomach cut open showing food material inside

other pyogenic infection or metastasis. Also try to find out by moving the loops of intestines for presence of any bullet or pellets in case of firearm injury after getting the X-ray of the abdomen done. Any foreign body found in the abdominal cavity should be duly preserved and handed over to the IO of the case. The intestines and stomach in case of suspected poisoning should be persevered for chemical analysis of poison. Colon should be looked for any mass or abnormal mucosa which should be sent for histopathological examination to rule out cancer. In case of cholera the rugae of the mucosa are lost. A typhoid/amebic ulcer, if any, should be distinguished. Typhoid ulcer is present longitudinally along the Peyer's patches and amebic ulcer is present transversely. The intestinal walls look paper-thin in case of starvation deaths.

Figure 15.8 shows congested organs in asphyxial death.

Removal and Examination of Kidneys

The soft tissues above and medial to the adrenal and kidney areas in the abdominal cavity are cut with a curved incision made towards the lateral abdominal wall. This is joined by another curved incision along the lateral border of the kidney to meet the superior incision. The incision should penetrate the peritoneum and perinephric fat. The hand of the autopsy surgeon is introduced into the hole, thus produced and the kidney along with the adrenal gland is grasped and attached soft tissues dissected all round except the medial part where the renal vessels and ureters are present. The renal vessels are examined for presence of any thrombi. Pelviureteric junction and ureter are examined for any calculus by dividing the ureter either high up or inferiorly along its length. The kidney along with adrenal is then removed after tying a thread to the ureter along with the vessels about 1 inch away from the hilum. Any atrophic or hypertrophic kidney should be noted.

Weight of normal adult kidney is about 150 gm.

The external surface should be examined for any congestion seen in most of the poisoning and asphyxia death cases, subcapsular hematoma, hemorrhage due to injury. The internal examination is done by making a longitudinal sagittal slice from the convex border of kidney using a brain knife. The slice is extended to the pelvis of the ureter through the parenchyma. The cut slice is then opened like a book (Fig. 15.6) and the cortex and medulla are assessed for any loss of corticomedullary demarcation which is commonly seen in

1. Renovascular hypertension,
2. Diabetes or
3. Chronic glomerulonephritis
4. Nephrosclerosis
5. Infection/septicemia due to trauma or systemic disease

The renal arteries should be examined for any stenosis or presence of thrombus. The renal pelvis and ureter are looked for presence of any calculus.

Postmortem report: After complete external and internal examination of a dead body, the findings are written/typed in a pre-designed proforma (enclosed) and report is prepared.

The final postmortem report in original is handed over to the investigating officer after obtaining receipt in the postmortem form itself and a copy is kept in the record of the forensic medicine department of the hospital.

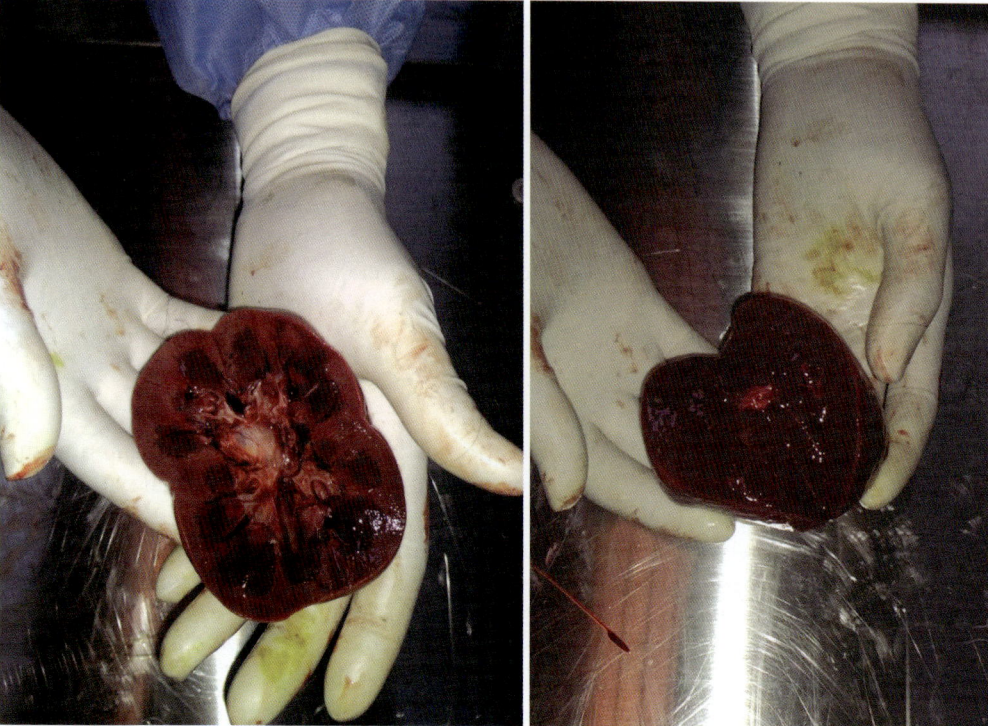

Fig. 15.6: Cut section of congested kidney

Fig. 15.7: Cut section of congested spleen

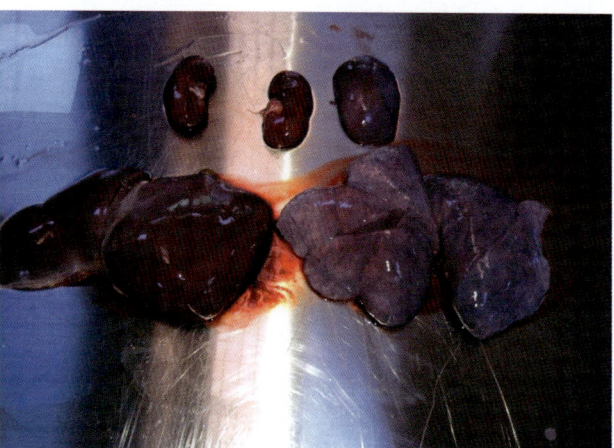

Fig. 15.8: Congested liver, spleen, kidneys and lungs in a case of asphyxia

MODEL POSTMORTEM REPORT FORM

विधि चिकित्सा विभाग
DEPARTMENT OF FORENSIC MEDICINE
Hospital with address ....

शव परीक्षण रिपोर्ट सं.
POSTMORTEM REPORT NO ....

शव एवम् जांच पडताल कागजात प्राप्त करने की तिथि व समय
Date & Time of receiving dead body and inquest paper _____

शव परीक्षण शुरू करने की तिथि व समय
Date & Time of starting autopsy _____

शव परीक्षण समाप्त करने की तिथि व समय
Date & Time of concluding autopsy _____

शव लाया व पहचाना गया
Body brought & identified by

1 जांच अधिकार का नाम/Name of Investigating officer_____ थाना / Police Station _____

2 कांस्टेबल/Constable _____ सं. / No. _____
शव पहचाना गया

Body also identified by
1 नाम व पता/Name & address _____

_____ मतक के साथ संबंध / Relation with deceased _____

2. नाम व पता/Name & address _____

_____ मतक के साथ संबंध / Relation with deceased _____

मृतक का नाम	पिता / पति	आयु	लिंग
Name of deceased_____	Father / Husband _____	age _____	sex ____

पता
Address _____

मामले का संक्षिप्त इतिवृत (जांच पडताल कागजातो के अनुसार)
Brief history of the case (As per Inquest Paper)

उँचाई/Height _____ भार/Weight _____

(क) सामान्य अवलोकन
(A) General observation

शव परीक्षण रिपोर्ट सं.
POSTMORTEM REPORT NO.: ....

(ख) बाह्य चोटों का विवरण

(B) Details of external injuries

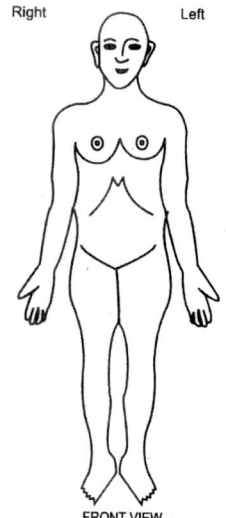

Right   Left

FRONT VIEW

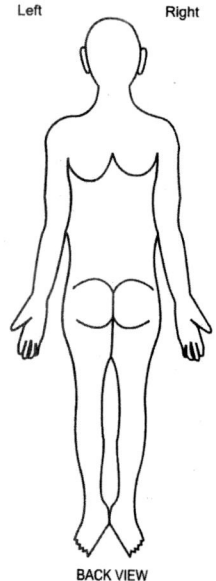

Left   Right

BACK VIEW

(ग) आन्तरिक परीक्षण

(C) Internal Examinations

1. सिर व गला / Head and neck

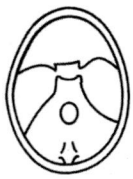

Right lateral   Left lateral
view   view

Base of skull

II छाती/Chest (Throax)

III पेट व अन्य/Abdomen and others

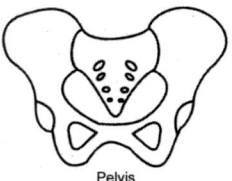

Pelvis

शव परीक्षण रिपोर्ट सं.

POSTMORTEM REPORT NO.: ....

(घ) रासायनिक विश्लेष्ण के लिए रखे गए सुरक्षित नमूने (यदि आवश्यक हो)

(D) Viscera preserved for chemical analysis during autopsy (if required) _____

(ड) परिरक्षी प्रयोग में लाया गया

(E) Preservative used: Saturated salution or common salt / rectified spirit any other _____

(च) कपड़े/अन्य सुरक्षित रखी गई वस्तुएं (यदि कोई हों)

(F) Clothes/other articles preserved during autopsy (if any) _____

(छ) टिप्पणियाँ (यदि कोई हो)

(G) Remarks (if any) _____

(ज) निष्कर्ष

(H) Opinion _____

चिकित्सा अधिकारी का पद नाम व हस्ताक्षर

Signature & Designation of Medical Officer

पुलिस को दी गई वस्तुएं :

Item handed over to police.

1. जांच पड़ताल के कागजात/Inquest papers _____ in numbers.

2. शव परीक्षण/Postmortem report in original

प्राप्तकर्ता पुलिस जांच अधिकारी का नाम   सं.   पुलिस स्टेशन

Name of receiving police investigating officer   No.   **Police Station**

हस्ताक्षर

Signature

Transplanted Kidney Examination

Transplanted kidneys are located in the pelvis connected with the iliac blood vessels. All the sutures in the kidney should be inspected before its removal. Vascular or ureteric anastomosis should be examined. Then the vessels are opened through the anastomotic sites to find out any intraluminal obstruction. The specific findings to look for in the transplanted kidney are infection, rejection and recurrence of glomerulonephritis, which sometimes require histological confirmation. Other features to look for are changes of chronic renal failure, cyst formation in dialysis cases. A recent complication is the emergence of post-transplant lymphoproliferative disorder. A block of such transplanted kidney tissue as well as the normal kidney tissue should be sent for opinion of a pathologist.

Examination of Female Genital Organ

Usually the uterus along with cervix, ovaries, fallopian tubes and upper vagina are removed together.

External Examination

The uterus normally measures 8 cm (long) × 6 cm (broad) × 4 cm (thickness of wall)

Weight of adult uterus is about 60–70 gm. Uterus is looked for any rupture, usually seen in illegal abortion or cesarean section by an unskilled doctor. Contusion due to blunt trauma, if any, should be noted. Uterus will be absent in cases of hysterectomy or congenital absence.

Internal Examination

Uterus is opened by a longitudinal cut from the vaginal cuff to the fundus through the cervix. This is done by introducing a probe through the external cervical os to corpus of uterus and cutting with a scalpel until the endometrium is exposed. This will help inspection of endometrium, myometrium and cervix. The midline incision is then extended to the uterine cornu and into the fallopian tubes. Thickness of uterine wall after cutting it should be measured. The uterine cavity is looked for presence of any pus, liquid or clotted blood, foreign body, fibroid, tumor or fetus. Fallopian tubes are inspected for tubal pregnancy, ligation, tumor, blood or pus. Cervical os if constricted in a full-term pregnant female leading to rupture of uterus should be noted. Vaginal introitus should be examined for any injury or *in situ* foreign body. Any foreign body found should be preserved along with the whole uterus with its contents if required.

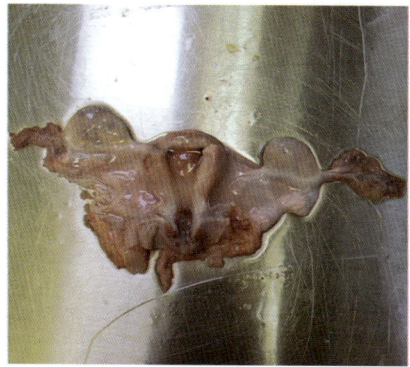

Fig. 17.1: Uterus, fallopian tube cut open by T-shaped incision showing the cavity

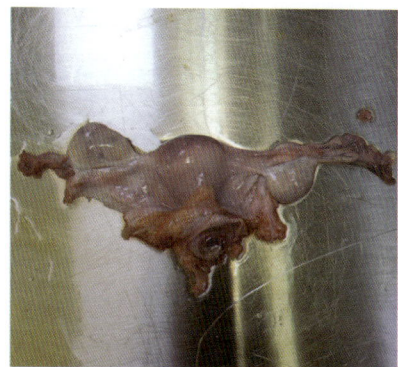

Fig. 17.2: Intact uterus, fallopian tube and ovary

Examination of Male Genital Organ

Both penis and scrotum should be inspected for any injury. Amputation of penis by a sharp object during an attempted rape or as revenge due to some other reason, laceration as seen in road traffic accidents. The scrotum should be looked for any bruise or lacerated injuries. Sometimes the testes are seen lying outside the scrotal sac in cases of accidents on road or railway track where the impact of the wheels are in the pelvic area. The testes can be lacerated or crushed by heavy blunt force trauma or explosion. It should also be looked for any tumor or ectopic testis.

Weight of each testis in adults is 12–14 gm.

Measurement is 5 × 3 × 2.5 cm.

Prostate Gland Examination

Prostate is the size of a walnut located between the penis in front and urinary bladder behind. The urethra runs through its center from bladder to the penis.

Size of adult prostate is about 20 gm in volume.

Measurement is 3 cm (L) × 4 cm (B) × 2 cm (Depth)

Prostate is inspected while opening the bladder during routine dissection of pelvic organs.

Transverse slices are made through the gland. Hyperplasia, if any, is noted. This organ can also be involved in blunt force trauma to the pelvis.

Fetal Medicolegal Autopsy

Before going into the details of autopsy the doctor should be conversant with the following definitions:
1. Embryo—product of conception from 1–8 weeks of gestation
2. Fetus—from 8 weeks of gestation to full term.
3. Neonate—from full term till one month after birth.
4. Infant—from one month till one year after birth
5. Infanticide—it is the unlawful killing of an infant below the age of one year.
6. Foeticide—it is the unlawful killing of a fetus any time before birth. For example: Illegal or criminal abortion.

Before postmortem the following clinical history either from the mother (in live birth) or from hospital record must be obtained:
1. Age, parity and ethnic origin of mother.
2. Gestational age at birth
3. History of any maternal illness
4. History of previous pregnancies terminating into dead born or stillborn fetus.
5. Details of present pregnancy like LMP, EDD
6. Details of labor and mode of delivery of the fetus.

In live born fetus:
1. Birth weight
2. Any resuscitative measures used in cases of respiratory distress or hemodynamic imbalance.
3. Neonatal course.
4. Childhood illness or congenital anomaly.
5. Details of death and preceding events
6. X-rays, CT scan or other imaging techniques used should be duly preserved.

All the above information helps the doctor in doing a meticulous postmortem with a proper technique. The formalities are the same as in an adult autopsy. The alleged fetus is brought by the police/investigating officer with an inquest paper requesting the doctor to conduct the autopsy on the fetus.

The objectives of fetal autopsy are:
1. Whether is it human fetus or not?
2. If yes, what is the intrauterine age of the fetus?
3. What is the sex of the fetus?
4. Is the fetus viable or not?

5. If viable, is it live born, stillborn or dead born?
6. How long did the fetus survive after birth?
7. Cause of death in live born fetus.

During medicolegal autopsy of fetus the opinion about the cause of death should be based on the postmortem findings falling under the following three categories:

1. *Live born fetus:* As per Indian Law—a fetus was alive after complete birth or when any part of its body comes out of the birth passage irrespective of the duration of gestation and who after such expulsion breathes or shows evidence of life.
2. *Dead born fetus:* A fetus which has died *in utero* long before labor. Dead born fetus shows the following sign after it is completely born:
   a. Maceration
   b. Rigor mortis
   c. Putrefaction
   d. Adipocere
   e. Mummification
3. *Stillborn fetus:* One who being born after 28 weeks of gestation did not breath or show any signs of life any time after being completely born (WHO). It was alive *in utero* but died during the process of delivery.
4. *Viable fetus:* It means a fetus which is capable of independent existence of mother after birth without attaining full term by virtue of certain degree of development. The age of viability varies from country to country anytime from 24 to 28 weeks of gestation. In India the age of viability has not been legally defined, however, medically it is taken as 28 weeks or 7 months of gestation.

Postmortem Examination of Fetus

Live Born: External

1. Clothes or wrappings, if any, should be noted.
2. Crown heel and crown rump length is measured.
3. Weight
4. Head circumference, chest becomes barrel-shaped after respiration increasing its circumference as compared to abdominal circumference at the level of umbilicus.
5. Umbilical cord length, whether torn or clamped at the stump or dried up cord. Drying occurs by 12 to 24 hours, inflammatory ring forms at the base by 36 to 48 hours and cord gets detached 5 to 6 days after birth.
6. Placenta whether attached with umbilical cord or not, infarcts, if any, are noted.
7. Any evidence of cyanosis, pallor, jaundice, edema and meconium staining should be assessed to rule out any physiological or disease condition of the fetus.
8. External injury in relation to obstetric and neonatal history, bruise, laceration in other body parts should be looked for which is usually seen in forceps delivery or in act of violence.
9. A search for petechial hemorrhages over the head, neck, chest and conjunctiva should be made. It is commonly seen in asphyxial deaths, e.g. smothering of the live fetus by the accused.
10. Any swelling in the fetal head because of collection of blood between the layers of scalp (caput succedaneum) or between periosteum and skull (cephalohematoma)

in cases of dilated cervix or forceps delivery respectively should be noted. Caput is a generalized or bilateral swelling seen in vertex presentation. It usually disappears by 1 to 7 days. Cephalohematoma is localized due to attachment of fibrous tissues between skull sutures. It never crosses the suture line. It is usually seen over the right parietal bone. The swelling increases during the first 2 days after birth and disappears by 6 to 7 weeks after birth.

11. Skin for initial 2 to 3 days is dark red or purple in color, then it becomes bright red and by 7th day it assumes the normal skin color.
12. Vernix caseous are looked for on the skin over the axilla, neck and inguinal folds of the fetus. It is a waxy or cheese-like white substance. It is composed of sebum, sloughed off fetal skin and shed lanugo hair. It persists for 1 to 2 days after birth. It does not always indicate live birth.

Before opening the body cavities ossification centers are examined to assess the age of fetus irrespective of live/still or dead born.

Demonstration of Ossification Centers

a. The knee joint is flexed against the thigh and a transverse incision is made in the front in bent of the joint. The soft tissues are reflected upwards and lower end of femur is exposed. Thin slices are made by a cartilage knife in **lower end of femur**. The ossification center is seen as reddish spot surrounded by bluish white cartilage. Same procedure is done for the **upper end of tibia.** These ossification centers are seen in the 9th month of intrauterine life or at birth.

b. For bones of foot a longitudinal incision is made on the sole of the foot from the space between 3rd and 4th toes to the heel. The lateral flap is then reflected exposing the outer border of the foot. The underlying calcaneum, talus and cuboid are then sliced in the sagittal plane to see their ossification. The calcaneum appears in the 5th, talus in the 7th and the cuboid in the 9th month of intrauterine life (IUL).

c. Sternum bone is placed on a wooden board and longitudinal cut is made in the midline with a cartilage knife exposing the ossification centers towards the cut end. Ossification for manubrium and 1st sternebrae appear at 5th month, 2nd and 3rd sternebrae at 7th month, 4th sternebrae at 10th month of IUL and xiphisternum at 3rd year after birth (Fig. 19.1).

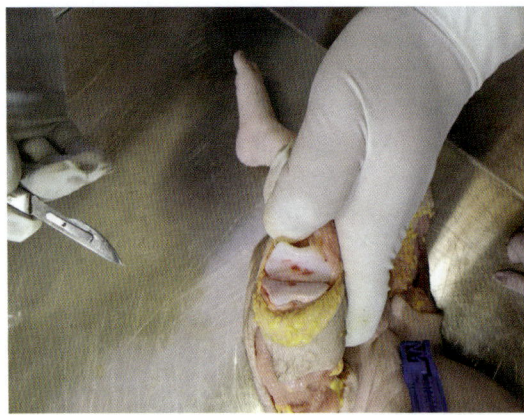

Fig. 19.1: Ossification center (red spot) at the lower end of femur of a 9-month-old fetus

Internal Examination and Opening of Body Cavities of Fetus

Skull: Steps

1. A coronal skin incision should be made well behind the ear in the occipital area of the fetal skull.
2. The posterior skin flap is then reflected back as far as the suboccipital region.
3. Sagittal incisions are then made parallel to and a little away from sagittal suture on both sides of midline starting from the coronal incisions in the occipital area already made.
4. The incision is then extended to the frontal area where it meets the 2nd coronal incision over the skin of frontal cartilage of the fetal skull. The 4 skin flaps are then opened like petals of a flower exposing the underlying cartilaginous fetal skull. The skull is opened by separating the frontal, coronal, sagittal and lambdoid sutures which exposes the underlying fetal brain (Figs 19.2 and 19.3).
5. Any subdural and subarachnoid hemorrhage should be looked for in the brain which can now be removed as in case of adult. Where the brain is soft, flabby or fragile it is better removed by lifting the feet of the fetus with one hand while the other hand is placed on the brain which is carefully kept on the dissecting table for complete examination.

Chest and Abdominal Cavity: Steps (Figs 19.4 and 19.5)

1. An inverted Y-shaped incision is made from the submental point to umbilicus which is then bifurcated on two sides of midline to the iliac fossae.
2. Pneumothorax as described in adult is checked.
3. Ribs are cut at the costochondral junction.
4. Sternal flap removed and chest cavity examined.
5. The level of diaphragm is assessed. Before respiration it is at the level of 4th or 5th rib. After respiration it is at the level of 6th or 7th rib because the inflated lungs push the diaphragm downwards.
6. Lungs are examined for whether or not respired.

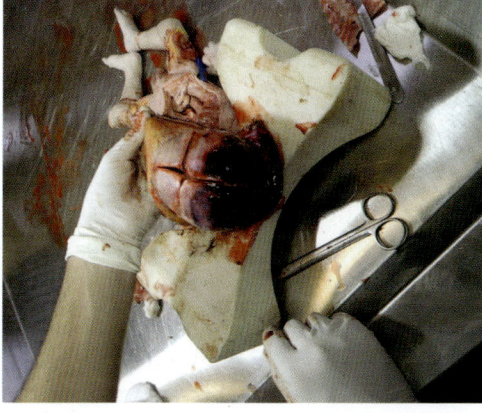 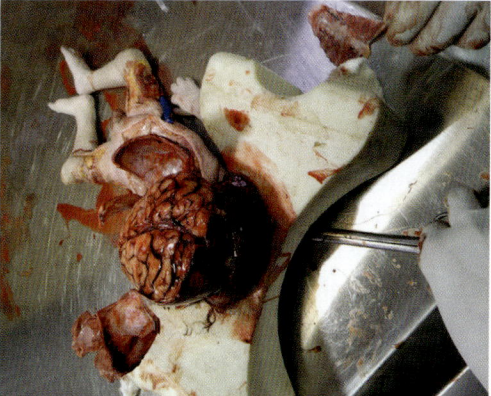

Fig. 19.2: Dissected fetal skull with caput over occipital region

Fig. 19.3: Brain after removal of fetal skull

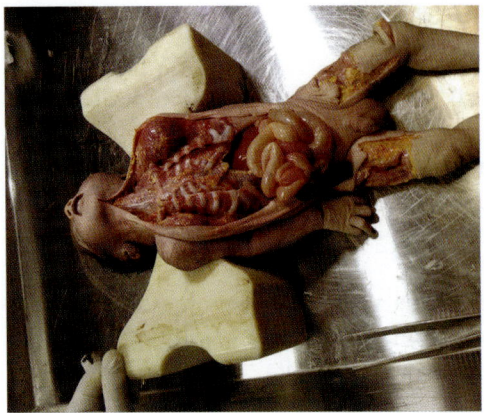

Fig. 19.4: Dissection of 9-month-old fetus

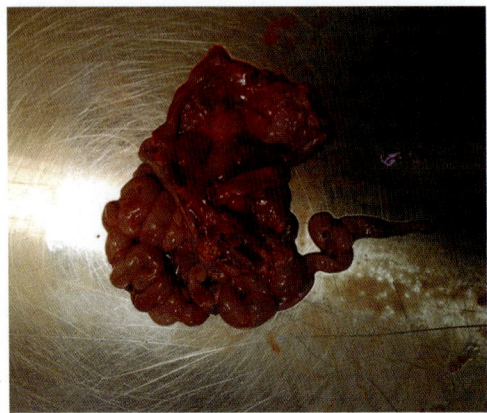

Fig. 19.5: Intestines stomach of a fetus

The following are the differentiating features:

Respired	Not respired
Color—mottled or marbled	Uniformly blue or violet.
Volume—large overlapping the heart	Small
Weight is 1/35th	1/70th of total body weight (Ploucquet's test)
Weight is 30 to 40 gm	60 to 70 gm (Foderre's test)
Margins are rounded	Sharp
Consistency is soft, spongy and crepitant	Liver like, hard and non-crepitant
Hydrostatic test is positive (floats)	Negative it sinks in water

This test is not required if the fetus is less than 180 days, macerated or mummified, monster fetus (developmental anomaly such as anencephaly), stomach contains milk.

False positive hydrostatic tests are observed in:
1. Putrefying gases in lungs
2. Attempted artificial respiration by pushing air into lungs

False negative hydrostatic test is observed in:
1. Atelectasis
2. Consolidation because of pneumonia.
3. Cut section of lungs shows abundant frothy blood /little frothless blood.

Maceration seen in a dead born fetus is a state of aseptic autolysis after its intrauterine death and has the following features:
1. A rancid (rotten, foul smelling oil or fat) odor is emitted from the fetus
2. The body flattens when kept on the table because of its pliability and softness.
3. All the joints are hypermobile.
4. The viscera, except lungs and uterus loose their morphology.
5. **Spalding's sign** which is overriding of vault of skull bone seen in radiograph due to shrinkage and liquefaction of brain matter inside the skull is positive when the fetus has died *in utero* between 5 and 7 days back. Maceration sets in 5–7 days before the birth of the fetus and takes about the same time to form.

6. Abdominal cavity is opened. All the abdominal organs are examined. The stomach and intestines are removed after tying with a double ligature at each end and then putting in water. If it floats, then the fetus has swallowed air and was live born, otherwise it will sink **(Breslau's second life test).**

   Meconium is a green colored viscid substance consists of inspissated bile and mucus which is expelled from colon within 24 hours after live birth.

7. Umbilical vessels are examined for any vital reaction which indicates survival from 24 to 48 hours after birth.

Stillborn fetus usually has the following external features
1. Edematous due to prolonged labor. May be absent sometimes.
2. Caput succedaneum may be present due to bleeding in the scalp.
3. Severe moulding of head due to difficult vaginal delivery.
4. Absence of maceration.

Internally the following features are seen in stillbirth
1. Gross pulmonary edema
2. Alveolar duct membrane is present and is evenly distributed in the lungs.
3. Atelectasis due to obstruction by alveolar duct membrane.
4. Pulmonary contusion (after excluding the hemorrhagic disease).

Causes of stillbirth are
1. Anoxia
2. Prematurity
3. Intracranial hemorrhage due to birth trauma
4. Toxemia of pregnancy
5. Congenital anomalies

   In spite of the above findings in most of the cases it is difficult to differentiate between stillborn and dead born fetus by postmortem alone.

Custodial Death

Definition

Death of a person occurring in the custody of police or prison. The following situations can lead to such deaths:

1. Police officer using physical force in an attempt to detain a person in the police station.
2. Lack of proper treatment by the custodian authorities when a person has sustained physical trauma or suffering from some illness.
3. The person trying to escape from the custody.
4. During interrogation of a person under custody using various methods of torture by the custodian officers.

   Some of the physical violence used by the police may be: Blunt trauma caused by the use of fist, arm, leg, point of elbow or use of weapons like truncheon (short thick stick carried by the police), riot sticks or butts of guns, traumatic asphyxia, arm-lock neck holds. All these can lead to potentially fatal injuries due to reflex cardiac arrest by vagal stimulation of carotid sinus, subarachnoid hemorrhage from vertebrobasilar artery damage.
5. When the accused under custody uses weapons in an attempt to kill the police officer who is forced to subdue him/her by using batons or firearm in extreme cases.
6. Where death has occurred during the transport of the accused from prison to the court.
7. Hospitalized accused who is already under custody of police.
8. Alcohol intoxication by the alleged accused poses various other problems such as violent aggression leading to above consequences. In acute alcohol poisoning (blood alcohol above 350–400 mg/100 ml) can cause respiratory depression, which if prolonged leads to coma and ultimately death. At low blood alcohol level the person might aspirate the vomitus causing asphyxial death. Under the influence of alcohol the person may fall on a hard surface because of ataxia leading to fatal head injury.
9. Suicide by hanging is not uncommon cause of custodial death.
10. The person may die from purely natural disease such as CAD because of the stress of being arrested and confined to jail. A terminally ill patient of cancer or disease of infective origin can also die in prison because of inadequate/ absence of treatment. History of any disease like diabetes, epilepsy, pancreatitis, asthma, MDR or XDR tuberculosis must be obtained from the relatives of the deceased.

National human rights commission (NHRC) has issued the following guidelines for cases of custodial deaths:

1. All such cases should be inquired by a District Magistrate.
2. Police officer or the magistrate should report to the commission (NHRC) about the occurrence of custodial deaths within 24 hours.
3. Rectal temperature using a rectal thermometer and development of rigor mortis should be noted by a trained police officer of the prison at the earliest at the scene of death which help assess the time since death during postmortem examination.
4. The body must be put in a special body bag with a zip during transportation.
5. Clothing should not be removed from the body either by police or any other person as they are required as a part of postmortem examination. The clothes need to be examined by the autopsy surgeon.
6. A model autopsy form prepared as per the recommendation of NHRC should be used while writing the postmortem report and not the usual autopsy form.
7. All cases of custody deaths should be videographed (arranged by the IO of the case) along with the voice of the doctor to avoid any tampering of the report. This is also in the interest of the doctor for transparency of the procedure without any suppression of the facts under pressure or influence.
8. In deaths due to alleged firearm injury the part of the body as required should be radiographed to locate the bullet/pellet.
9. Still photographs with and without clothes, front, back, profile views with zooming on the injuries over the dead body should be taken. Photographs of the palm and sole after making incision are taken so as to reveal an underlying bruise caused by police beating. All the photographs should bear the postmortem number, date, and scale for dimension of injuries. Total photographs may be 20–25 in number.
10. Postmortem examination of custodial death is conducted by a panel of doctors either from one hospital or one doctor each from different hospitals being the members of the panel.
11. The inquest papers, postmortem report, cassettes of the video and photographs should be put in a sealed packet and sent to NHRC either directly by the doctor or through the investigating officer of the case. The enquiry of custodial death is conducted by session's judge and the police officer is prosecuted where a prima facie case has been established.

Postmortem Examination of Custodial Deaths

A meticulous postmortem should be done to prove or disprove the involvement of the police official in the death of the prisoner.

The clothes of the deceased should be thoroughly examined for tear, blood or other stains and any other findings elsewhere which is of importance for the case.

External Examination

- **The head** is examined by giving a coronal incision and bringing the front and back of the skin flap of the scalp up to the face and occipital protuberance respectively.
- **Front of the body** is examined by giving a modified Y-shaped incision.
- **Back of the body** is examined by a paramedian incision from occipital protruberance up to sacrum. The right and left skin flaps are then dissected laterally. Any injury to

the cervical and other vertebrae, back of ribs and contusion on the back of the body will be revealed. Both front and back of the body, head, neck, legs, hands, palm, sole of feet, axilla and genitalia should be examined for any contusion, abrasion, laceration and sometimes firearm injuries. Deep incision on the sole and palm reveals underlying bruise which may not be obvious on gross examination as the skin is thick. Majority of the injuries are contusion. The extent of contusion in the entire body surface should be precisely noted. Extensive contusion (bruise) can lead to circulatory collapse and death because of the decreased circulatory blood volume. Wherever necessary radiographs should be taken of the part of the body to find out any fracture of bone or missile of a firearm.

Internal Examination

This is mainly required to rule out coronary artery disease (CAD), rupture of enlarged spleen, liver, kidneys due to disease, contusion of viscera, rupture of Berry's aneurysm and vagal inhibition.

Allegations are brought against the police by the relatives of the prisoner although the cause of death is one of the natural diseases listed above. The opinion about the cause of death in custody should not be revealed to the police as investigating officer of custodial death is a Magistrate.

Model Postmortem Report Form (NHRC)

Name of Institution ....

Postmortem Report No. .... Date ....

Conducted by Dr. ....

Date and time of receipt of the body and inquest papers for autopsy ....

Date and time of commencement of autopsy ....

.... Time of completion of autopsy ....

Date and time of examination of the dead body at inquest (as per inquest report)

....

In alleged encounter deaths, it may be done in scientific manner along with still photography.

Case Particulars

1. (a) Name of deceased as entered in the Jail or Police Record ....

   ....

   (b) S/O, D/O, W/O ....

   (c) Address: ....

2. Age (Approx): .... yrs; Sex: Male/Female

3. Body brought by (Name and rank of police officials)

   (i) ....

   (ii) .... of

   Police Station ....

4. Identified by (Names & addresses of relatives/acquaintance)

   (i) ....

   (ii) ....

5. If death occurred in hospital (particulars as per hospital records)
   Date and time of admission in hospital ....
   Date and time of death in hospital ....
   Central Registration no. of hospital ....
6. Alleged history (in brief, as per inquest papers)

Schedule of Observations
A. General
1. Height .... cm
2. Weight .... kg
3. Physique:
   a. Lean/medium/obese
   b. Well built/average built/poor built/emaciated
4. Identification features (if body is unidentified)
   i. _____
   ii. _____
   iii. Fingerprints be taken on separate sheet and attested by the doctor.
5. Description of clothes worn—important features:
6. Postmortem (PM) changes:
   • PM staining/lividity
   • Rigor mortis (if present, the extent)
   • Decomposition changes (if any)
7. External general appearance
   a. Condition of eyes
   b. Natural orifices (mouth, nose, ears)
   c. Nail

B. External Injuries: (Mention type, shape, length × breadth × depth of each injury and its relation to important body landmark. Indicate which injuries are fresh and which are old and their duration.)
   i. Injuries be given serial number and mark similarly on the diagrams attached.
   ii. In stab injuries, mention angles, margins and direction inside body.
   iii. In firearm injuries, mention about effects of fire also.

C. Internal Examination
1. Head
   a. Scalp findings
   b. Skull (describe fractures here and show them on body diagram enclosed)
   c. Meninges, meningeal spaces and cerebral vessels (hemorrhage and its locations)
   d. Brain findings and Wt. (_____gm)
2. Neck
   • Mouth, tongue and pharynx
   • Larynx and vocal cords
   • Condition of neck tissues
   • Thyroid and other cartilage conditions

3. Chest
- Ribs and chest wall
- Esophagus
- Trachea and bronchial tree
- Pleural cavities—R .... L ....
- Lungs findings and wt—R .... gm and L .... gm
- Pericardial sac
- Heart findings and wt .... gm
- Large blood vessels

4. Abdomen
- Condition of abdominal wall
- Peritoneum and peritoneal cavity
- Stomach (wall condition, contents and smell) (weight .... gm)
- Small intestines, appendix
- Large intestines and mesenteric vessels
- Liver including gall bladder (wt .... gm)
- Spleen (wt .... gm)
- Pancreas
- Kidneys finding and wt—R .... gm and L .... gm
- Bladder and urethra
- Pelvic cavity soft tissues
- Pelvic bones
- Genital organs (Note the condition of vagina, scrotum, presence of foreign body, presence of fetus, semen or any other fluid, and contusion, abrasion in and around genital organs).

5. Spinal Column and Spinal Cord (to be opened where indicated)
6. Additional remarks, if any, only.

Opinion
  i. Probable time since death (keep all factors including observations at inquest)
  ii. Cause and manner of death: The cause of death to the best of my knowledge and belief is:
    a. Immediate cause
    b. Due to
    c. Which of the injuries are antemortem/postmortem and duration if antemortem?
    d. Manner of causation of injuries
    e. Whether injuries (individually or collectively) are sufficient to cause death in ordinary course of nature or not?
  iii. Any other

Specimens Collected and Handed Over (Please tick)

a. Viscera (stomach with contents, small intestine with contents, sample of liver, kidney (one half of each), spleen, sample of blood on gauze piece (dried), any other viscera, preservative used)

b. Clothes

c. Photographs (video cassettes in case of custody deaths, fingerprints, etc.).

d. Foreign body (like bullet, ligature, etc.).

e. Sample collected for histopathological examination (mention name of organs/tissues).

f. Sample of seal

g. lnquest papers (mention total number and initial them)

h. Slides from vagina, for semen or any other material.

Postmortem report in original, ... inquest papers, dead body, clothings and other articles (mention there) duly sealed (Nos. ....) handed over to police official .... No. .... of PS .... whose signatures are herewith.

Signature: ....

Name of Medical Officer ....

(in block letters) ....

Designation ....

SEAL

DNA Profiling

Applications, sample collection and preservation.

The following are the applications of DNA profiling:

1. Paternity and maternity establishment
2. Personal identification
3. Identification of criminals involved in homicide or rape from biological evidence left at the scene of crime
4. In cases of child swaping
5. In organ transplantation to match donor and recipient
6. Identification from mutilated body parts in cases of mass disaster.
7. Identification from skeletal remains
8. To detect bacteria and other organisms that may pollute air, water, soil and food.

As per CDFD (Center for DNA Fingerprinting and Diagnostics, Hyderabad), the following guidelines are supposed to be observed:

- For establishment of maternity/paternity disputes, blood stains of the mother, disputed child and the alleged/suspected biological father is required.
- For identification of rapist in sexual assault cases, the following articles, viz. garments, vaginal swabs and slides along with the blood stains of the suspect(s) and victim are required.
- For identification of dead, blood stain of nearest relatives (viz. mother, father, brother, sister and children are required along with material object of the deceased like teeth, postmortem blood, muscle tissue, bone, hair with root and other material relevant to the case).

Following samples should be collected from living subjects for DNA profiling

1. **Blood**—obtained from veins or capillaries
2. **Buccal epithelial cells**—from inside the cheeks using sterile swabs. Two swabs—one each from inside of right and left cheeks. It should be dried at room temperature and should not be put in any container.
3. **Hair follicles**—between 10 and 15 hairs should be pulled with roots from the subject.

Following samples should be collected from a dead body

1. **Blood stain**—wrapped with a dry paper or cloth
2. **Muscle tissue**—about 100 gm of muscle tissue in a clean glass bottle/plastic container with 0.9% normal saline on ice or in a crystal salt on ice or in a crystal salt (sodium chloride) as preservative. It should never be preserved in formalin.

3. **Vaginal swabs**—the dry cotton swab should be placed in a clean, dry glass bottle/vial.
4. **Teeth, hair with root and bone (intact)**—wrapped in a dry paper or cloth

Samples to be preserved from a charred (burnt) dead body
1. Skeletal muscle from deep regions of body, like thigh, gluteal region or any area with incomplete charring.
2. Semisolid blood that remains inside cardiac chambers.

Samples to be preserved from a decomposed and skeletonized body
1. Long bone preferably femur or any bone with intact bone marrow
2. Teeth—after dental charting at least 4 teeth preferably molars wherever possible.

All the above samples should be duly sealed, along with a sample seal and handed over to the IO for transfer to the CDFD.

Completely burnt bones and decomposed tissues are not useful for DNA analysis.

Toxicology

Toxicology

Forensic Toxicology

Forensic toxicology is a branch of science which deals with the study of medicolegal aspects of deleterious effects of various poisons on human body. The following definitions are of importance in understanding the subject.

Toxicology: Refer to definition in chapter 2 on page 4.

Toxinology is a branch of science which deals specifically with the study of biological toxins such as venoms, plants, bacteria, fungi and animals.

Poison: Poison is any substance solid, liquid or gaseous which if comes in contact with or administered by any route to human body will cause ill effect or death by its local, systemic or effects combined.

IPC Sections in Relation to Poisoning

Laws in Relation to Toxicology in India under Indian Penal Code

Sections (IPC) Descriptions

1. 176: Doctor should report all cases of homicidal poison to police for magisterial inquiry.
2. 193: Doctor is punishable for giving false information of a case of poisoning. Punishment—7 years imprisonment and fine.
3. 284: Causing harm to anybody through rash and negligent handling of a poison. Punishment is imprisonment up to 6 months with or without fine.
4. 299: Culpable homicide by any means including poisoning.
5. 300: Homicide by any method including poison.
6. 304A: Rash and negligent act by any means including poison. Punishment is up to 2 years or fine or both.
7. 324: Causing hurt by dangerous weapon or means including poison. Punishment is up to 3 years or fine or both
8. 326: Grievous hurt by dangerous weapon or means including poison. Punishment is up to 10 years or life imprisonment with or without fine.
9. 328: Causing hurt by means of poison with the intention to commit an offence. Punishment is up to 10 years imprisonment and fine.
10. 326A: Punishment for throwing of acid or corrosive on a person is imprisonment for 10 years.

Duties of a Doctor in
Case of Poisoning

Primary (professional) duty of a doctor is to save the life of the patient followed by the legal duties.

The professional duties include:

1. The patient should be removed immediately to a place away from the source of poison, particularly in case of inhalation poison to fresh air.
2. For injectable poison a ligature should be tied proximal to site of injection/bite which is loosened every 10 minutes to prevent gangrene formation to the affected part of the body.
3. In contact poisoning the part should be thoroughly washed with water or any neutralizing agent.
4. In ingested (oral route) poison should be removed from the body before the poison is absorbed into the system by stomach wash or emesis.
5. Type of poison consumed should be detected, if possible.
6. Depending upon patient's condition attention should be paid to maintain airway, breathing and circulation (ABC).
7. Supportive treatment should be started at the earliest.

Legal duties of a doctor in case of poisoning are:

1. In a government hospital every case of poisoning (accidental/homicidal/suicidal) should be reported to the police.
2. In a private set-up suicidal poisoning may or may not be reported. But it is better to report such cases as well.
3. All cases of suspected/definitive homicidal poisoning should be reported by the physician to the police under Sec. 39 Cr. Pc. Failure to do so will make the doctor culpable under Section 176 IPC.
4. If the doctor deliberately withholds or gives wrong information in a poisoning case, the doctor becomes culpable under Sections 202 IPC (deals with intentional omission of information and is punishable with imprisonment up to 6 months) and 193 IPC (giving false evidence and is punishable up to 7 years of imprisonment).
5. Doctor should collect the gastric lavage, vomitus, urine, faeces as evidence of the alleged poisoning subject. Any deliberate attempt not to collect them may attract a punishment under Section 201 IPC (punishment for causing disappearance of evidence with up to 7 to 10 years of imprisonment).
6. If the victim is on the verge of death, the doctor should inform the magistrate to record a dying declaration of the dying person at the earliest or treating physician can also record it if the arrival of magistrate is delayed.

7. If the patient dies during the course of treatment or was brought dead, death certificate should not be issued and the local police should be informed to make arrangement for postmortem examination.
8. Doctor should maintain a detailed written record of all cases of poisoning.
9. Doctor should certify that the victim is conscious and mentally fit to give statement of the circumstances leading to his present condition.
10. In cases of food poisoning the doctor should collect the food sample for chemical/ analysis by Forensic Science Laboratory and should also report about such cases to the public health department.

Preservation of Viscera in Poisoning Cases

In almost all cases of alleged poisoning body organs and tissues need to be preserved for qualitative and quantitative analysis of alleged poison.

The common preservatives used are:

1. Saturated solution of common salt, prepared by adding common salt in water till the salt remains undissolved even after thorough stirring. This preservative is used in most of the poisoning cases.
2. Rectified spirit is used in most of the poisons, except alcohol, phosphorus, carbolic acid, acetic acid, kerosene, etc. In alcohol poisoning 125 mg of sodium fluoride is added in 25 ml of blood. Potassium oxalate is used as an anticoagulant in other poisons. In gaseous or volatile poisoning a thick layer of 2–3 cm of liquid paraffin is added over the blood sample to prevent evaporation of the gaseous/volatile poison.

Some of the common viscera and tissues preserved in all cases of poisoning are:

1. Stomach (whole of it), small intestines (proximal 30 cm) with their contents.
2. Liver—minimum 500 gm along with the gall bladder.
3. Spleen—whole of it
4. Kidneys—half of each kidney.
5. Blood—10–20 ml of venous blood.
6. Urine—total quantity available in the bladder.

Some special organs and tissues preserved in special cases of poisoning are:

1. Brain—one cerebral hemisphere or 500 gm. In cases of CNS and volatile poisons, e.g. barbiturates, carbon monoxide, cyanide, opiates, alcohol, anesthetic agents.
2. Spinal cord—entire length in cases of strychnine poisoning
3. Lungs—half of each in cases of inhalation poisoning sent in air-tight container.
4. Heart—whole of it in case of cardiac poisoning
5. Muscle—200 gm. In case of putrefied organs.
6. Bones—long bone, preferably femur (10 cm length) in case of heavy metal poisoning.
7. Scalp hair—plucked along with the root in cases of heavy metal poisoning.
8. Nails—all nails in cases of arsenic poisoning.

Classification of Poisoning

Poisons have been classified by various ways. Most commonly used classification is based on the mode of their action. The following are the six major groups:

A. Corrosives (Caustics)

1. *Strong acids*
   a. Mineral (inorganic) acids: For example: H_2SO_4, HCl, HNO_3 (Fig. 26.1)
   b. Organic acids, e.g. carbolic, acetic and oxalic acid
2. Strong alkalies, e.g. ammonia, caustic potash, caustic sodium, carbonates of sodium and potassium.

B. Irritants

1. *Inorganic*
   a. Metallic (heavy metals): For example, arsenic, lead, copper, mercury, zinc, antimony, thallium (Fig. 26.2)
   b. Non-metallic, e.g. phosphorus, chlorine, iodine (Fig. 26.4)
2. *Organic*
   a. Irritant plants, e.g. castor, croton, calatropis, abrus (Figs 26.4 and 26.5)
   b. Animals, e.g. snake, scorpion, spider, bee, wasp, cantharides

C. Neurotics

Cerebral
a. Somniferous, e.g. opium and opiates (Figs 26.3 and 26.7).
b. Inebriants, e.g. alcohol, barbiturates, benzodiazepines
c. Deliriants, e.g. datura, cannabis, coccain (Figs 26.3, 26.6 and 26.8).
d. Psychotropic:
   1. Hallucinogens, e.g. LSD, phencyclidine
   2. Neuroleptics (antipsychotics), e.g. olnazepine, queitiapin, risperidone, etc.
   3. Antidepressant, e.g. TCAs, MAOIs, SSRIs (selective serotonin reuptake inhibitors)
   4. Spinal—e.g. nux vomica, gelsemium (Fig. 26.3)
   5. Peripherally acting—e.g. curare, Conium maculatum (hemlock).

D. Cardiac

For example, aconite, oleander, digitalis, nicotine, hydrocyanic acid (Figs 26.3 and 26.4).

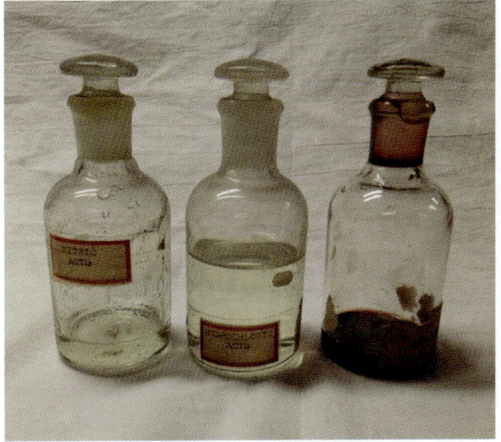

Fig. 26.1: Corrosives H_2SO_4, HCl and HNO_3

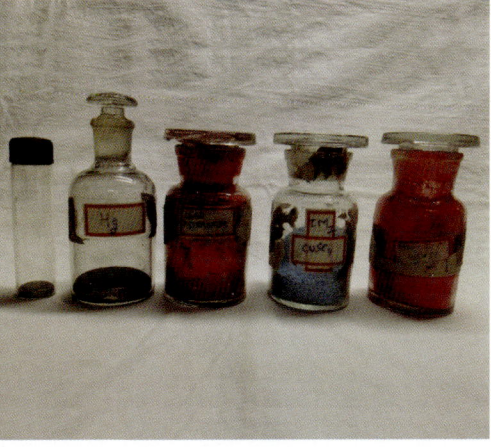

Fig. 26.2: Metallic poisons. Mercury metal, salts of lead, copper and mercury

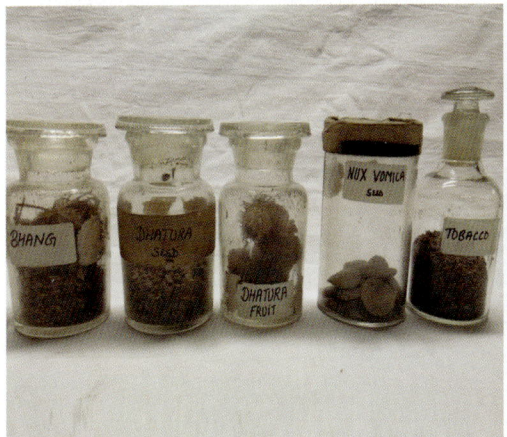

Fig. 26.3: Neurotic poisons. Bhang (cannabis leaves) opium (poppy fruit), *dhatura* fruit, nux vomica seed and tobacco leaves (cardiac)

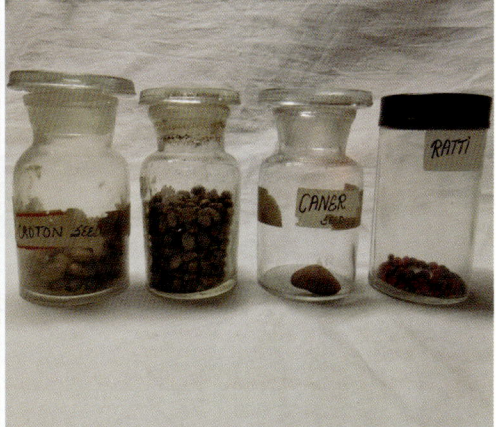

Fig. 26.4: Vegetable irritants and cardiac poison croton seeds, castor seeds, kaner (cardiac), ratti seeds

E. Aphyxiants

For example, carbon monoxide (CO), carbon dioxide (CO_2), hydrogen cyanide (H_2S), methyl isocyanide, methane, tear gas, war gases.

F. Miscellaneous Poisons

1. Agrochemicals, e.g. insecticides and pesticides
2. Food poisoning, e.g. bacterial (botulism), fungal (mushroom), chemicals
3. Substance of abuse, e.g. hallucinogens, sedatives, antidepressants
4. Petroleum products, e.g. kerosene, petrol.
5. Pharmaceutical products, e.g. analgesics, antipyretic, antibiotics, tranquilizers

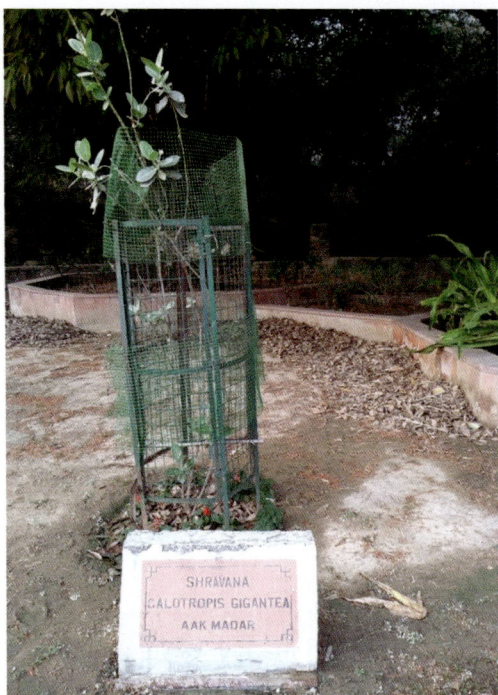

Fig. 26.5: Calatropis (madar) plant

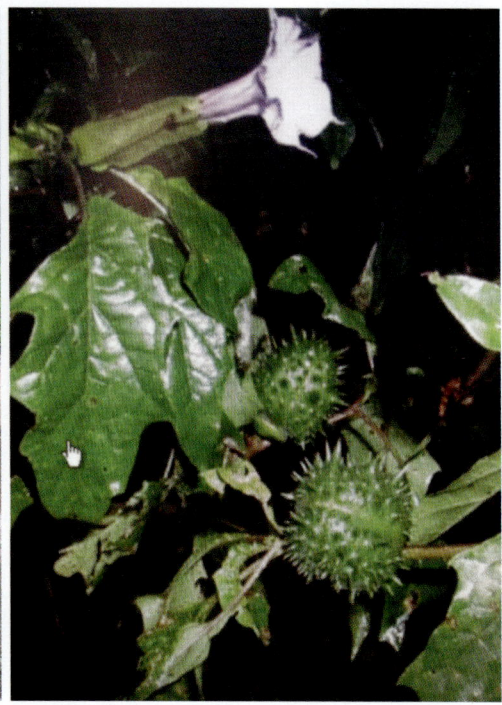

Fig. 26.6: Datura leaf, flower and fruit

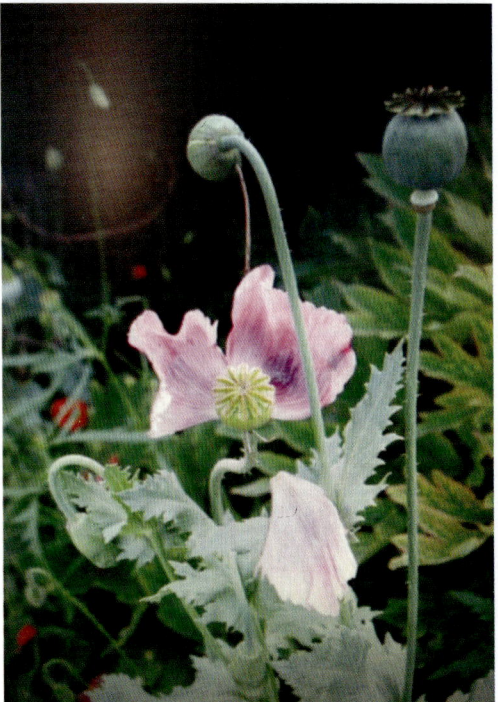

Fig. 26.7: Poppy plant with flower and fruit (opium is obtained from unripe fruit)

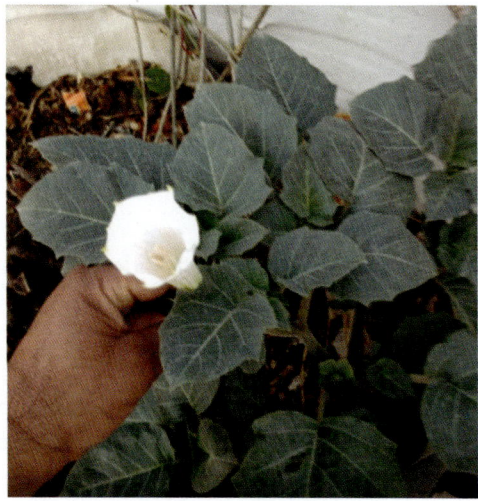

Fig. 26.8: Datura flower

Individual Poisons—Signs, Symptoms and PM Findings

Any case of suspected poisoning is a medicolegal case. However, some of the important and common poisons will be dealt with in subsequent chapters from the point of view of:

1. Identification of the poison
2. Signs and symptoms of poisoning and
3. Postmortem findings in the event of death.

Corrosives

SULFURIC ACID

It is also known as oil of vitriol. It is a heavy, colorless, viscid/oily, non-fuming liquid. It produces heat with water and causes charring when come in contact with human tissue.

Signs and symptoms on oral ingestion are:
- Severe burning sensation and pain from mouth till the stomach.
- Dribbling of acid mixed saliva from angle of mouth causing corrosion over the skin till its flow.
- Oral mucosa and lips are excoriated with blackish discoloration of necrotic tissue.
- Teeth are chalky white due to loss of polished enamel.
- Intense thirst, vomiting and dehydration
- Voice is hoarse and husky due to inflammation of epiglottis
- Some signs of asphyxia due to edema of glottis.
- Constipation and tenesmus
- Perforation of stomach and intestine is rare
- Stomach is blackened with a peppery feel
- Corrosion and inflammatory changes are present in the trachea and larynx.

Cause of death
- Immediate—asphyxia due to edema of glottis, circulatory collapse due to dehydration.
- Delayed due to starvation as a result of esophageal and pyloric stricture.

Postmortem findings
External—Corrosion of body parts that come in contact with the acid.
Internal—Findings are restricted to the upper GIT and respiratory tract. Pharynx and esophagus show inflammatory changes with bleeding and edema. Larynx and trachea show corrosion and inflammation.
Fatal dose—10 to 15 ml
Fatal period—12 to 24 hours.

HYDROCHLORIC ACID

It is a colorless fuming liquid with a pungent odor. Because of its volatile nature it mainly affects the respiratory tract.

Signs and symptoms: Since it is less strong than sulfuric and nitric acid, it does not cause corrosion of skin. Inhalation of fumes may cause irritation of upper respiratory tract with symptoms of cough, respiratory distress.

Cause of death: Same as for sulfuric acid.

Postmortem findings
Almost same as for sulfuric acid except that charring is less.
Fatal dose—15 to 20 ml.
Fatal period—18 to 24 hours.
Cause of death: Same as for sulfuric acid.

NITRIC ACID

It is a colorless fuming heavy liquid when fresh, but older samples have yellowish tint.

Signs and symptoms: When comes in contact with human skin, it causes xanthoproteic reaction, a yellow discoloration because of its combination with tyrosine protein present in skin and mucus membrane.

When the fumes are inhaled it will cause cough, dyspnea, intense irritation in pharynx and lungs. Lacrimation if fumes come in contact with eyes.

Postmortem findings: Same as sulfuric acid with minimal charring and tissue destruction.

Cause of death: As for sulfuric acid.
Fatal dose—10 to 15 ml
Fatal period—12 to 24 hours.

CARBOLIC ACID (PHENOL)

It is a colorless needle like crystals. It turns pink and liquefies when exposed to air. Commercial carbolic acid is dark brown liquid. Coal tar, thymol and menthol are some of the derivatives of phenol. Mostly used as disinfectant, antiseptic and germicide.

Signs and symptoms
- On local application it acts as a corrosive with necrosis and sloughing with whitish eschars.
- It damages the nerve endings, therefore, causes numbness with no pain.
- On ingestion there is burning sensation in the mouth and throat.
- Headache, giddiness, tinnitus
- Pain abdomen
- Hypothermia and hypotension are sometimes present.
- Carboluria is seen if the victim survives for 48 hours. when there is renal damage with scanty urine which is dark colored. On exposure to air the urine becomes olive green in color because of the presence of metabolites of phenol, viz. pyrocatechol and hydroxyquinone.
- Ochronosis the pigmentation of cornea, veins, cartilages due to the presence of above two metabolites. Usually seen in chronic poisoning.

Postmortem findings
- Dark brown excoriations around angle of mouth
- Tongue is swollen and whitish in color

- Characteristic odor of phenol comes out from oral cavity.
- Esophagus has grey white, corrugated mucosa
- Stomach is described as "leather bottle stomach" with hard mucosa.

Therefore, this is the only corrosive poison where stomach wash can be done as there is no chance of perforation.

Cause of death: Asphyxia due to edema of glottis and respiratory failure. Shock due to circulatory collapse.

Fatal dose—10 to 15 gm or ml

Fatal period—3 to 4 hours

OXALIC ACID (ACID OF SUGAR)

It is a colorless, odorless, prismatic crystal with a sour taste. It is used as an ink remover, stains on clothing, and writings on cheque/paper for forgery.

Signs and symptoms
- Locally it produces yellowish corrosion on skin or mucus membrane (oral ingestion).
- Vomiting
- The color may be blackish if acid hematin is formed.
- Coffee colored vomiting and diarrhea
- Tetany due to hypocalcemia characterised by muscle spasm, cramps. Positive Trousseau's sign (fingers of hand undergo a spasm) and Chvostek's sign (muscles of face show twitching when facial nerve is tapped).
- Cause of death—shock
- Acute renal failure
  Fatal dose—15 to 20 gm
  Fatal period—1 to 2 hours

  Postmortem findings:
  - Yellow or whitish discoloration of corroded mucosa of mouth, lips and tongue.
  - Stomach contents are brownish, mucosa is punctate and reddish due to erosion, wall is soft without any perforation.
  - Kidneys are congested and enlarged, tubules are filled with oxalate crystals.
  - Rest of the viscera shows congestion.

STRONG ALKALIS

Most of them are available either as white powders or colorless liquids, e.g. domestic cleaning agents, soap manufacturing industries. Ammonia is a colorless gas with a pungent smell.

Signs and symptoms
- When ingested it causes burning sensation inside mouth and throat.
- Vomiting, hematemesis, abdominal pain, diarrhea and tenesmus.
- Greyish, soapy and necrotic area without any charring are seen when it comes in contact with skin
- Inhalation of ammonia fumes causes respiratory symptoms.

Postmortem findings
- The mucosa of esophagus is corroded with greyish pseudomembrane formation.
- Stricture of esophagus is more common in alkali poisoning than acid.
- Congestion of GIT
- Corrosion and sliminess of the affected tissues

Fatal dose

10 to 15 gm for most of the alkalis

15 to 20 ml of ammonia liquid and 0.5% in air in gaseous form.

Alkali poisoning is more dangerous than acids as it produces liquefactive necrosis resulting in penetrating damage because of saponification of fats and dissolving the protein of the tissues.

Cause of death: Same as other corrosive agents.

AMMONIA

It has a characteristic pungent odor. Available as ammonium hydroxide liquid or ammonia gas.

Signs and symptoms
- Inhalation causes breathlessness, cough, watering from nose and eyes.
- Ingestion causes severe pain in upper GIT, vomiting, dysphagia
- Contact dermatitis if involves skin
- Corneal damage and conjunctivitis if involves eyes.

Postmortem findings
- Characteristic pungent odor from the body
- Greyish sloughing of affected body part.
- Congestion of viscera.
- Congestion of respiratory tract with pulmonary edema.
- Cause of death: Bronchopneumonia, pulmonary edema.

Potassium carbonate (caustic soda), sodium carbonate (washing soda) and potassium hydroxide (caustic soda): These alkalis are available as white crystalline powder and are soluble in water. They are used as cleansing agent in washing powder and blocked pipes.

Signs and symptoms

On ingestion there is burning sensation in the mouth and esophagus with an acrid taste. Vomitus and stool contains altered blood.

Postmortem findings

The entire GIT shows corrosion with patchy dark brown areas. The stomach content is blood stained.

Cause of death: Hemorrhagic and hypovolemic shock

Fatal dose
- Potassium carbonate (caustic soda): 18 gm
- Sodium carbonate (washing soda): 30 gm
- Potassium hydroxide (caustic potash): 5 gm

Irritants

METALLIC IRRITANTS (Fig. 10.2)

1. Arsenic (Sankhyal)

It is a heavy metallic inorganic poison. The metal is not poisonous, but its salts like arsenic oxide and arsenic trioxide are poisonous. The other salts like arsenic trihydride (arsine gas), arsenic trichloride, lead arsenate, copper arsenite are used in various industries.

Signs and symptoms: On ingestion there is metallic taste, dysphagia, vomiting, rice water diarrhea (similar to cholera), oliguria, uraemia, convulsions. Transverse opaque bands on nails (Mee's lines), loss of hair.

Postmortem findings
- Rigor mortis lasts longer
- GIT congested with red velvety stomach and sometimes flea-bitten appearance due to focal hemorrhage.
- Intestines inflamed and contain rice water like liquid.
- Subendocardial hemorrhage
- Fatty degeneration of liver and kidney.
- As arsenic is radiopaque, X-ray of abdomen may show its presence in the intestines.

Cause of death—hypovolemic shock
Fatal dose
100 to 200 mg for arsenious oxide
200 to 300 mg for arsenic trioxide
Fatal period—2 to 3 days.

2. Lead (Shisha)

It is a soft, steel-grey colored heavy metal used in various industries like paint, glass, plastics, enamel wares, batteries, welding and in some ayurvedic medicines. The various lead salts are lead acetate (sugar of lead), lead carbonate (white lead), lead tetroxide (vermilion or sindur).

Signs and symptoms: Acute poisoning is rare, which could be exacerbation of chronic poison. In chronic poisoning (plumbism) there is
- Facial pallor
- Anemia (microcytic, hypochromic)
- Reticulocytosis

- Punctate basophilia (basophilic stipplings in RBC)
- Burtonian line (lead line), a stippled blue line seen at junction of gums particularly in carries teeth of the upper jaw (due to deposition of lead sulfide)
- Lead colic in abdomen, constipation (dry bellyache)
- Lead palsy due to paralysis of extensor muscle of finger (wrist drop)
- Lead encephalopathy
  Fatal dose—depends upon the salt, for lead acetate it is 20 gm
  Fatal period—1 to 2 days.

Postmortem findings

In acute poisoning
- Skin and conjunctiva is pale.
- GIT mucosa is congested, eroded with patchy greyish white deposits

In chronic poisoning
- Large intestines contain black colored stool.
- Intestines are thickened and contracted.
- Blue line over gum.
- Kidneys, liver contracted
- Heart hypertrophied

3. Mercury (Para, quick silver, liquid metal)

It is a heavy liquid metal with silvery luster and is volatile at room temperature. Some of its poisonous compounds are:
- Mercuric chloride (corrosive sublimate)
- Mercurous chloride (calomel)
- Mercuric sulphide (cinnabar, vermillion or sindoor)
- Mercuric oxide (sipichand)

Poisoning with mercury compound is commonly seen in the following industries:
- Thermometer manufacturing
- Barometer manufacturing
- Electrical appliances, e.g. mercury bulbs, thermostat.
- Ceramics
- Electroplating

Signs and symptoms
- Metallic mercury is not poisonous.
- Poisoning are commonly seen with mercuric chloride and mercurous chloride compounds.

Acute poisoning
- On ingestion there is acrid metallic taste, hoarse voice and difficulty in breathing, abdominal pain, burning sensation from esophagus to stomach, vomiting of greyish slimy material with streaks of blood, gingivitis, necrosis of jaw.
- Renal tubular and glomerular necrosis
- Peripheral blood smear will show leukocytosis.

Chronic poisoning
- On ingestion metallic taste, excessive salivation
- A blue line on the gums (Burtonian line) is seen
- Mercurial tremor which first appears in the hand leading to change in handwriting as it first affects the fingers, then progresses to lips and tongue causing stammering and slurring of speech, ultimately involves the arms and legs. The tremors are coarse with jerky movements. This tremor is called Hatter's shake as mercury was used in hat industry for giving a particular kinking shape to the felt hat (a hat that protects the head from bad weather and has brim all around)
- Mercuria lentis is a brownish deposit of mercury on the anterior lens capsule when viewed through a split lamp. It causes visual disturbance.
- Erethism is a cognitive disorder consisting of irritability, timidity, amnesia, insomnia, delusion, hallucination, bouts of anger, depression, sometimes leading to insanity (mad hatter).
- Acrodynia (pink disease): It is a condition where there is erythematous, eczematous papular rash seen in hands and feet due to prolonged exposure to mercury in any form.

  Fatal dose

  1–4 gm of mercuric chloride.

  10–60 mg/kg of methyl mercury. 10 mg/mm^3 of mercury vapor

  Fatal period—3–5 days

Postmortem findings
- Mucus membrane of oral cavity shows diffuse greyish white escharotic appearance.
- Stomach and intestine show corrosion and ulceration. Caecum, colon and rectum may become gangrenous if patient survives for a few days.
- Liver shows fatty generation
- Kidneys show tubular necrosis

NON-METALLIC IRRITANTS

Phosphorus

It is an irritant, inorganic, hepatotoxic protoplasmic poison. It exists in two forms—
a. White or yellow phosphorus
b. Red phosphorus

White phosphorus occurs as waxy, translucent, white soft sticks. It is insoluble in water and soluble in alcohol.

Red phosphorus is obtained by heating white phosphorus at 250°C with nitrogen or carbon dioxide.

Uses
1. It was used in manufacture of friction matchsticks, but because of risk of chronic poisoning it has been withdrawn. Present safety matchstick contains potassium chlorate and antimony sulfide.
2. In military uses yellow phosphorus is an ingredient of incendiary bomb, tracer bullet, smoke screen

3. Insecticide and rodenticide—it is an ingredient of powder and pastes used for killing cockroaches and mice.

Signs and symptoms
The symptoms appear 2–6 hours after ingestion

Primary phase
- Garlic taste in mouth and smell in the breath.
- Burning sensation in mouth, throat, epigastrium, phosphorescent vomitus and stool. Stools sometimes emanate fumes, a phenomenon called smoky stool syndrome.

Secondary phase
There are no symptoms in this phase and the patient feels normal which may last up to 2–4 days.

Tertiary phase
In this phase the poison is absorbed into the system. All the symptoms of primary phase reappear with increased intensity along with the effect of hepatotoxicity. Jaundice, pruritus, bleeding from multiple natural orifices. Ultimately hepatic encephalopathy develops leading to coma and death.
Fatal dose: Adult—60–120 mg
Children—10–25 mg
Fatal period—4–7 days

Postmortem findings
External—hemorrhagic patches under the skin. Dried/liquid blood at natural orifices. Phossy jaw may be observed in chronic phosphorus poisoning. It is the periostitis and osteomyelitis of the jaw along with necrosis of the alveolar part of mandible resulting in sloughing of gum and falling of teeth.

Internal
- On opening the abdominal cavity there is a garlicky odor except in decomposed bodies.
- The GIT is inflamed with yellowish/greenish stain.
- Liver is enlarged (sometimes shrunken in acute yellow atrophy), yellowish, soft, fatty degeneration with necrotic changes.
- Other organs also show fatty degeneration.
- Viscera preservation—phosphorus is never preserved in rectified spirit as it is soluble in alcohol.

Neurotics

SOMNIFEROUS POISON

Opium (Afim)

Botanical name is *Papaver somniferous* (Poppy plant) (Fig. 10.7). The plant grows everywhere in India. Cultivation of this plant is restricted and requires a license from the Government of India. A government opium factory is situated in Gazipur district of Uttar Pradesh. Unripe fruit capsule (Poppy) yields the toxic juice which is obtained by giving multiple parallel vertical incision on its surface. Opium is the dried form of the juice. When fresh opium is reddish brown, coarsely granular hard mass. Opium is an alkaloid.

The seeds present inside the fruit are edible and known as khas-khas. The various derivatives of opium are:

Natural
1. Morphine—a white crystalline powder with bitter taste, soluble in alcohol or water.
2. Codeine— same as morphine, soluble in water only.
3. Thebaine—Appear as prismatic crystals
   Natural and semisynthetic derivatives of opium are called opiates.
4. Heroin (diacetylmorphine) or brown sugar (semisynthetic)
   Synthetic derivatives of opium are called opioids (Fig. 10.3).

Synthetic
1. Dionin (ethylmorphine)
2. Pethidine
3. Methadone
4. Pentazocine

Signs and symptoms
a. Stage of excitement—euphoria, hallucination and convulsions especially in children
b. Stage of stupor—weakness, headache, giddiness, desire to sleep, itching of skin, constricted pupil (pinpoint pupil).
c. Stage of narcosis—patient goes into a stage of deep coma, pinpoint pupil, conjunctival congestion, hypotension, muscles relaxed, reflexes absent, Cheyne-Stokes breathing, respiratory arrest and death.

Fatal dose
Crude opium: 2 gm
Morphine: 180–480 mg

Codeine: 800 mg
Pethidine: 1 gm
Metadone: 100 mg
Pentazocin: 300 mg

Postmortem findings

External

- Emaciated, dirty clothes and body, sometimes long bearded and untidy scalp hair.
- Injection prick marks, abscess and old scars are seen over cubital fossa, dorsum of hands or other parts of body.
- Froth around mouth and nostrils
- Phlebitis and sclerosis of veins of upper limbs

Internal

- Trachea wall congested with presence of froth
- Lungs are congested and edematous with patchy hemorrhage.
- Right ventricular hypertrophy
- All organs are congested and edematous
- Lumps of opium may be found in the stomach content if crude opium has been ingested. Stomach wall is congested.

DELIRIANT POISON

Datura (*see* Figs 26.6 and 26.7)

It is one of the three groups of cerebral poison belonging to the vegetable deliriant type. Botanical name of the plant *Datura fastuosa*. The fruits are spherical with sharp spines all over and are called Thorn Apple.

It is found in wastelands almost everywhere.

Active principles are alkaloids:

a. Hyoscine (scopolamine)
b. Hyoscyamine
c. Atropine (causes symptoms of toxicity)

Signs and symptoms

On ingestion of seeds, symptoms appear within half an hour. The signs and symptoms are because of the anticholinergic effect of atropine and can be described in the form of 10 Ds as follows:

1. Dysphagia—because of inhibition of salivation
2. Dysarthria—because of inhibition of salivation
3. Dilated pupil
4. Diplopia—because of dilated pupil
5. Dry hot skin—as a result of inhibition of sweat secretion and dilatation of cutaneous blood vessels.
6. Dermatitis
7. Delirium—pill-rolling/muttering/threading an imaginary needle because of its effect on CNS
8. Drunken gait—same reason as in '7' above
9. Drowsiness
10. Death due to respiratory failure.

Fatal dose—100–125 datura seeds (500 mg–1 gm), 30–50 datura seeds cause stupefaction, 120 mg of atropine. 30 mg of hyoscine

Fatal period—24 hours

Postmortem findings: Nothing specific. Signs of asphyxia are present—all the organs are congested, lungs are edematous Datura seeds may sometimes be found in the stomach.

INEBRIANT POISON

1. Alcohol

Details of clinical aspects and signs and symptoms have already been described.

- It is important to know that after death ethanol is spontaneously produced in the body because of the action of enzymes, bacteria, yeast or fungi on proteins and carbohydrates on putrefied body. Therefore, the postmortem analysis of viscera may show a high level of alcohol even in a person who has not consumed alcohol prior to death. However, such postmortem alcohol level will not exceed 50 mg%.
- After death, alcohol diffuses through the stomach to pericardial, pleural and peritoneal fluid and surrounding tissues. Therefore, after death the blood sample for alcohol estimation should not be drawn from the area surrounding the stomach as it will give false high level of alcohol.
- Ideally postmortem blood should be collected from femoral or cubital vein.
- The concentration of blood alcohol after death is reliable for a period of 36 hours after death.
- Postmortem vitreous humour and urine are quite reliable samples for estimation of blood alcohol level before death.
- When the person is in the stage of coma (6th stage) after alcohol consumption (BAC 300–500 mg%) and does not recover even after 5–6 hours, death is likely due to shock or asphyxia.
- Death is very rare after consumption of pure ethanol.
- Sudden death after alcohol consumption is possible as it predisposes to cardiac arrhythmia because of interaction of catecholamines with alcohol especially during/ after struggle or fight.

  Fatal dose—150–250 ml of absolute alcohol or 6 gm/kg body weight (in non-addicts)

  Fatal period—12–24 hours, may be delayed up to 5 days.

2. Barbiturates (goofballs, pink, barbs)

- Barbiturates are derivatives of barbituric acid
- They are used as sedative or hypnotic, usually administered orally (as tablets), intravenously (as liquid). Barbiturates are classified as—ultra-short acting (action lasts for <15–20 minutes), short acting (action lasts for <3 hours), intermediate acting (action lasts for 3–6 hours), long acting (action lasts for 6–12 hours).
- Barbiturates when mixed with alcohol is dangerous as the CNS depressant effect of both is potentiated. A little overdose of this combination is usually fatal. Intravenous injection of it is a common method of suicides among doctors who are easily accessible to these drugs.

Signs and symptoms
- Drowsiness
- Confusion, delirium, hallucination
- Ataxia, vertigo, slurring speech
- Headache
- Level of consciousness depressed to a varying degree
- Pupils are initially constricted but becomes dilated in the terminal stage
- Babinski reflex is positive
- Hypothermia and hypotension
- Cutaneous bullous (barbiturate blisters) formation seen in 6–10% cases with intermediate acting barbiturates
- Barbiturate automatism is a condition where the person takes more and more of the drug for relief from some pain unknowingly that he/she has already taken a dose, this leads to overdosage and ultimately death.
- Respiratory rate reduced as it depresses the medullary center. There is Cheyne-Stoke's breathing in the terminal stage ultimately leading to death due to respiratory failure.

Fatal dose—long acting: 3–4 gm, intermediate acting: 2–3 gm, short acting: 1–2 gm, ultra short acting: 1.5–2 gm

Fatal period—24–48 hours.

Postmortem findings
- Features of asphyxia in the form of cyanosis of face and nail.
- Traces of tablets may be found inside the mouth, esophagus or stomach
- The mucosa of stomach is congested and eroded.
- Lungs are congested and edematous.
- Petechial hemorrhage are present on the pleura, pericardium and meninges.
- Subendocardial hemorrhage in acute barbiturate poisoning.
- Kidneys are congested with changes of degeneration.
- Brain is congested and edematous with petechial hemorrhage

3. Benzodiazepines

They are used as anxiolytic, sedatives, hypnotics, muscle relaxant and anticonvulsants. Death by benzodiazepines alone is very rare. However, death has been reported in elderly persons with flunitrazepam, diazepam, alprazolam, flurazepam.

Signs and symptoms

Acute poisoning: Weakness, amnesia, diplopia, ataxia, slurred speech and vertigo.

Chronic poisoning: Tolerance develops, withdrawal symptoms characterized by headache, insomnia, anxiety, tremors, convulsion and psychosis.

Fatal dose: They are safe drugs and rarely cause death. Cases have been reported where persons have survived even after taking 30 to 50 times the therapeutic dose. Postmortem findings—nothing specific. Depends on the organ involved.

Cardiac Poison

1. Hydrocyanic Acid (Cyanogen)

It is widely found in many leaves and fruits of plants such as peaches, plums, apricort, bitter almond in the form of a harmless glucoside known as amygdalin. The enzyme emulsion of these plants can hydrolyse amygdalin in presence of water to form hydrocyanic acid. Cyanide in the liquid form is called hydrocyanic acid and in gaseous form is known as hydrogen cyanide (HCN).

- Pure hydrocyanic acid is colorless, transparent volatile liquid with a peculiar odor of bitter almond. About 20–40% of the population is unable to smell the gas because of a sex-linked recessive trait.
- Cyanide salts of sodium and potassium are available as white powder.

Signs and symptoms
- On inhalation the action is immediate, within 1–2 minutes. On oral ingestion the symptoms of cyanide poisoning are delayed up to 15–20 minutes.
- On inhalation the person will have headache, giddiness, confusion, agitation, convulsion, loss of muscle power and unconsciousness ultimately leading to coma and death.
- On oral ingestion there will be burning taste with a sense of constriction and numbness in the throat, excessive salivation from the mouth. Frothing around the mouth with corrosion of the mucosa may be seen. Smell of bitter almond from mouth and in the breath.

Fatal dose
Pure hydrocyanic acid: 60 mg
Potassium cyanide: 200–300 mg
Air concentration of hydrocyanic acid: 1:500—immediate death.

Fatal period
Hydrogen cyanide inhalation: 2–3 minutes.
Potassium cyanide: About 30 minutes.

Postmortem findings
External
- Smell of bitter almonds near the body
- Rigor mortis sets early and lasts longer
- Fine froth in and around the mouth
- Eyes are bright, glistening and prominent with dilated pupil

- Postmortem staining is cherry-red color due to formation of cyanmethemoglobin
- Irregular pink patches over face and other parts of body.

Internal
- Odor of bitter almond on opening the body
- Trachea contains bloody froth
- Stomach mucosa is pink or crimson red in color
- Corrosion of mouth in potassium cyanide poisoning
- Lungs are edematous, pleura and pericardium may show petechial hemorrhage.
- All organs are congested.
- Blood is cherry-red color due to formation of cyanmethemoglobin.

Viscera to be preserved: Blood, stomach with its content, lungs, liver, spleen, heart, kidneys, brain. Spleen is the best organ to be preserved for detection of cyanide as it contains abundant RBCs with a very high concentration of the poison.

2. Nicotine (Tobacco)
- The plant usually grows in tropical countries.
- Botanical name is *Nicotiana tobacum*.
- The dried leaves of the plant contains the active principle—nicotine and lobeline. Nicotine is more toxic of the two.
- Nicotine is an alkaloid
- The dried leaves of tobacco plant are used for smoking. The leaves contain 1–8% of nicotine.
- The leaves are used variously for smoking, snuff, chewing. Tobacco when mixed with lime is called khaini.
- Nicotine content of a regular size cigarette is 13–20 mg, cigar is 15–40 mg. During smoking a substantive amount of nicotine remains in the butt and filter, some escape as side stream smoke, it is only about 1 mg of nicotine that finally enters the lungs.
- The smoke inhaled from a single cigarette decreases the oxygen availability to the tissues by about 8% because production of COHb.
- Nicotine itself is not carcinogenic but it is the tar which is produced by burning of tobacco is carcinogenic.
- In India bidis are smoked among the poorer section of society. They contain tobacco wrapped in a tendu leaf. Bidis are more harmful than cigarettes as they contain high nicotine, carbon monoxide and tar.

Signs and symptoms
Acute poisoning
- It occurs when tobacco leaves are chewed and manifested as nausea, vomiting, headache, giddiness, weakness, cardiac arrhythmia. After a few hours the person becomes normal.
- Toxicity from smoking has all the above manifestations with convulsions and delirium.
- Pupils are initially constricted, then become dilated.
- Death though rare may occur due to cardiac failure.

Chronic poisoning
- Besides cigarette smokers it is also seen in nicotine insecticide sprayers. It is manifested as chronic cough, bronchitis, laryngitis, pulmonary emphysema.
- Nicotine is an addictive substance and withdrawal symptoms are commonly seen. The manifestations are headache, anxiety, fatigue, insomnia, palpitation, tremors, nervousness and cramps.

Risk of following diseases increase manifold in tobacco smokers
1. Coronary artery disease (CAD)
2. Oral cancer
3. Lung cancer
4. Peptic ulcer
5. Hypertension, cardiac arrhythmias (ventricular fibrillation)
6. Optic atrophy
7. Thromboangiitis obliterans with symptoms of intermittent claudication.

Fatal dose—2 gm of tobacco or 60 mg of nicotine.

Fatal period—5 minutes–6 hours.

Postmortem findings
- Smell of tobacco on opening the stomach. Brownish discoloration with hemorrhagic patches of stomach wall
- All the organs are congested.

Asphyxiants

CARBON MONOXIDE (CO)

It is a colorless, odorless, non-irritating gas produced when there is incomplete combustion of carbon such as wood, charcoal, kerosene. Fuels of motor vehicle, automobile exhaust, tobacco smoke are other sources of CO. In the blood CO combines with hemoglobin and forms a stable compound carboxyhemoglobin. Hemoglobin has 200–300 times more affinity to carbon monoxide than oxygen.

Hemoglobin therefore becomes incapable of delivering oxygen to the tissues leading to tissue anoxia.

Signs and symptoms:
Stages: Depending on COHb percentage in blood.

Mild (COHb <30%)—throbbing headache, dizziness, dyspnea, irritability, nausea and vomiting.

Moderate (COHb 30–40%)—blurred vision, mental confusion, increased dyspnea, ataxia, tachycardia, dilated pupils, bullous formation over pressure areas of skin. Severe (COHb>40%)—severe headache, all the above symptoms are intensified, muscle spasm, disorientation, tachycardia, Cheyne-Stokes breathing, respiratory paralysis, coma. COHb> 80% leads to rapid death from respiratory failure.

Fatal dose and period

Concentration of CO gas in air (%)	Death (in hours)
1. 0.02%	4 hours
2. 0.04%	1 hour

Postmortem findings
- Cherry red coloration of postmortem lividity (appreciable in fair complexioned person), lips, fingertips.
- Frothing around mouth and nostrils
- Lungs are congested and edematous
- Anoxic necrosis of skeletal and myocardial muscles.
- Brain is edematous and shows punctate hemorrhages in globus palladium and corpus striatum.

Sample/viscera preserved: Blood from peripheral vein. Sodium fluoride used as preservative and the bottle is sealed with a layer of liquid paraffin to prevent evaporation of CO.

Miscellaneous Poisons

AGROCHEMICALS

Insecticides

They are used as aerial spray, liquid or dusting powder on plants and soil.

Classification of Insecticides

1. **Organophosphates**, e.g.
   a. Alkyl phosphate, e.g. hexaethyltetra phosphate (HETP), tetraethyl pyrophosphate (TEEP), octamethyl pyrophosphoramide (OMPA)
   b. Aryl phosphate, e.g. parathion, diazinon, paraxon, chlorothion
2. **Organochlorides**, e.g. DDT, aldrin, endrin. The above classification of insecticide has been replaced by modern classification as follows:
   • Highly toxic (agricultural)—parathion, OMPA, TEEP, etc.
   • Moderately toxic (animal)—trichlorfon, ronnel
   • Mildly toxic (household)—malathion, diazinon (Tick-20)

Organophosphorus compounds: They inactivate the enzyme acetylcholinesterase resulting in accumulation of acetylcholine at the nerve endings. They are basically cholinesterase inhibitor. Therefore, they exhibit both muscarinic and nicotinic effects on the peripheral and central nervous system in the body.

Signs and symptoms: Muscarinic effects are manifested as breathlessness due to bronchospasm, increased salivation, bronchial secretion, lacrimation and sweating, tightness feeling in the chest, tenesmus, constricted pupils. Sometimes there is shedding of red tears due to accumulation of porphyrin in the lacrimal gland, a condition called chromolacryorrhea. Nicotinic effects are manifested as weakness, involuntary twitching of muscles with cramps, fasciculation, dyspnea due to effect on respiratory muscles, tachycardia, hypertension, cardiac arrhythmia, pulmonary edema, depression of respiratory and circulatory centers leading to coma and ultimately death.

Cause of death: Respiratory failure. In non-fatal cases patient recovers in 36–48 hours.
Fatal dose—malathion and diazinon 1 gm oral.
   OMPA—175 mg oral/80 mg injectable IM.
   Parathion—100–175 mg oral/80 mg IM.
   TEPP—100 mg oral/50 mg IM.
   Fatal period—symptoms start within half an hour and death occurs between 3 and 6 hours.

Postmortem findings
• Cyanosis of lips, nails
• Blood-tinged froth around mouth and nostrils

- Kerosene like smell on opening the body particularly from GIT
- Stomach mucosa is congested with petechial hemorrhages
- Lungs congested and edematous with hemorrhagic patches
- Brain congested, edematous and petechial hemorrhages
- All other organs are congested as in death due to asphyxia

CARBAMATES

They are similar to organophosphates but instead of permanent they temporarily bind cholinesterase enzymes for about 6 hours without any permanent damage to the tissues. They have poor CNS penetration and therefore CNS symptoms of carbamates are minimal. Signs and symptoms are similar to organophosphate. *Examples:* Sevin (carbaryl), Baygon (apocarb), Furaxdan (carbofuran).

CHLORINATED HYDROCARBONS OR ORGANOCHLORIDES

Examples are—endrin, aldrin, lindane (gamaxene), DDT (dichlorodiphenyl-trichloroethane)—they are commonly used as insecticide in agriculture and sanitation to kill bedbugs, flies, lice and other arthropods. They are a crystalline powder with an aromatic odor, soluble in organic solvents and insoluble in water. They are used in liquid or powdered form.

Signs and symptoms
After ingestion of the poison:
- Nausea, vomiting, abdominal pain.
- Giddiness, tinnitus
- Blurred vision, twitching of eyelids.
- Convulsion: Tonic and clonic type
- Dyspnea, pulmonary edema.
- Hypotension
- Unconsciousness, coma

Cause of death—Respiratory failure

Fatal dose
- DDT—30 gm or 0.5 gm/kg body weight
- Lindane (Gamaxene)—15 gm

Postmortem findings
- Stomach and intestines are congested with hemorrhagic patches.
- Kerosene like smell in the stomach contents
- Lungs are congested and edematous
- Liver enlarged with fatty degeneration
- All other organs are congested.

Pesticides

a. Fumigants, e.g. aluminum phosphide, dibromo-chloropropane, formaldehyde
b. Rodenticides (rat poison), e.g. zinc phosphide, warfarin, thallium, strychnine chlorphacinone, diphacinone

c. Herbicide (weed killers)—e.g. paraquat, glyphase
d. Moth repellent—e.g. napthalene

FUMIGANTS

a. Aluminium Phosphide

It is a grain preservative available in tablet form. It is sold in the market by the following names: Alphos, sulphas, celphos, fumigrain, quickphos. A single greyish color tablet weighs 3 gm. Each tablet releases 1gm of phosphine (PH_3) gas when comes in contact with water or acid which is poisonous to insects, rodents. Phosphine gas is a colorless gas but has a garlicky (fishy) odor.

Signs and symptoms
- When tablets are consumed by human being for committing suicide or by accidental inhalation of phosphine gas, it causes symptoms of GIT irritation, ARDS (acute respiratory distress syndrome), severe pulmonary edema. It also affects the heart causing cardiovascular collapse.
- There is burning pain in the epigastrium with nausea and vomiting
- Garlicky (fishy) odor from the breath
- Constriction feeling in the chest
- Cardiac arrhythmia
- Hypocalcemia tetany

Cause of death
- Cardiac failure (due to arrhythmia) within 24 hours of ingestion.
- Metabolic acidosis and respiratory alkalosis after 24 hours of ingestion.

Fatal dose: 150–500 mg (1 tablet) orally >400–600 ppm in air is fatal within half an hour of inhalation.

Fatal period—1–3 days.

Postmortem findings
- Frothing around mouth and nostrils in some cases
- Cyanosis of lips, fingers
- Garlicky smell on opening the body from gastric contents
- All the organs are congested with petechial hemorrhage
- Lungs are congested and edematous

b. Paraquat

It is widely used herbicide used as spray for removal of weeds which destroy the crops. It is available either as granules or odorless brown liquid. It is inactivated by the soil, therefore does not destroy the underground planted seeds. The weeds are killed as it is absorbed by the foliage. It is therefore used before planting any crops in the field. Paraquat is available by trade name Weedol, Gramaxone, Dextrone, Spot Killer, Cyclone.

Signs and symptoms
- On ingestion there is erosion of the mucus membrane of lips, mouth, esophagus. In extreme case it can cause perforation of GIT.
- On regurgitation of liquid it affects the lungs. The lungs are edematous and voluminous, sometimes weighing up to 2 kg.
- It is causes hepatic and renal toxicity with associated clinical symptoms.

Cause of death—hepatic or renal failure.

Fatal dose—4–5 mg/kg body weight

Fatal period—72 hours–7days depending upon the amount consumed.

Postmortem findings
- Ulceration around lips and mouth with desquamation of oral mucosa
- Lungs will be heavily edematous with indentations of ribs on the surface as seen in wet drowning cases. This type of lung is called paraquat lung.
- Liver will have a mottled appearance. Histopathology reveals centrilobular hepatic necrosis.
- Histopathology of kidneys shows acute tubular necrosis.

NAPTHALENE (TAR, CAMPOR)
- It is a moth repellent used for preservation of woolens and as lavatory deodorant.
- It is insoluble in water but soluble in ether and alcohol. It volatizes at room temperature.
- Napthalene is available in form of white scaly powder or as mothballs.

Signs and symptoms
- Vomiting, diarrhea, abdominal pain, convulsions.
- Burning micturition, hematuria, oliguria, hemoglobinuria, urine contains albumin. Napthalene causes hemolysis which blocks the renal tubules by precipitation of hemoglobin which is responsible for the above signs.
- Liver may show necrotic changes on histopathology.

Cause of death—acute renal failure.

Fatal dose—2–5 gm

Fatal period—within 72 hours

Postmortem findings
- Blood tinged froth around mouth, nostril, larynx and trachea.
- GIT is congested with a yellowish tinge
- Liver is congested and enlarged
- Kidneys are congested, cortico-medullary differentiation is indistinct.

Food Poisoning

WHO defines food poisoning as diseases, usually either infectious or toxic in nature, caused by agents that enter the body through ingestion or food.

Bacterial food poisoning are caused by presence of bacteria or their toxins in food. *Bacterial food poisoning are caused by*

1. *Clostridium botulinum*
2. Salmonella and Shigella
3. Staphylococcus
4. *E. coli*
5. Proteus

Nonbacterial food poisoning are caused by poisonous

a. Plants
b. Animals
c. Chemicals

Poisonous plants are

1. *Argemone mexicana* (satyanashi)
2. Lathyrussativus (khesari)
3. Cotton seeds
4. Mushroom (Khumbi, a fungus)

Poisonous animals are

1. Poisonous fish
2. Mussel (belong to molluscs family)

Chemicals

1. Coloring agents
2. Flvoring agents
3. Preservative

Bacterial food poisonings are

a. *Infective type:* In this type there is ingestion of live microorganisms which multiply in the GIT. Example: **Shalmonella and Shigella.**
b. *Toxic type:* In this type bacteria release enterotoxin which leads to poisoning. Example: **Staphylococcus.**

BOTULISM

The bacteria *Cl. botulinium* multiplies in food such as sausages, tinned food.

Signs and symptoms
- Vomiting with abdominal pain
- Constipation
- Ptosis
- Dilatation of pupil and diplopia
- Dysphagia, dysphonia
- Bilateral ascending motor neuron paralysis beginning with abducens (VI) or oculomotor (III) nerve palsy
- Urinary retention
- Respiratory distress
- Mental state, sensorium, reflexes, pulse and body temperature are usually normal.

Cause of death: Respiratory failure. Salmonella food poisoning are commonly seen when large amount of food is prepared but consumed after 2 or more days as in restaurants, hostels, canteens. Depending upon body resistant some person remain asymptomatic while others develop severe GI symptoms. The incubation period of this food poisoning (6–72 hours) is longer than that caused by Staphylococcus (30 minutes to 6 hours).

In Staphylococcus food poisoning there is:
a. Muscle palsy/weakness
b. Fever
c. Foul smelling diarrhea are absent, which differentiates it from Salmonella food poisoning. The organisms can be isolated by culture of the suspected food consumed

Postmortem findings
- Gastric and intestinal mucosa is congested and hemorrhagic.
- Histopathology of liver shows fatty degeneration.

MUSHROOM
- These fungi usually grow in moist areas.
- Amanita species are common.
- Active principle is Phalloidins

Signs and symptoms
Symptoms appear after 6–12 hours of ingestion in the form of
- Severe diarrhea, vomiting and abdominal pain
- Fever

Fatal dose—one full size mushroom

Fatal period—72 hours to one week.

Postmortem findings
- GIT is congested
- Hepatic and renal tubular necrosis on histopathology.
- Brain congested; substantia nigra may show necrotic changes.

LATHYRUS SATIVUS (KESARI DAL)

It is a type of dal consumed by villagers of North India. Prolonged consumption leads to poisoning called lathyrism.

Active principle—a neurotoxin BOAA (B oxalyl amino-L-ananine) that affects the pyramidal tract of the nervous system.

Signs and symptoms
- Pain in calf muscles
- Weakness of the legs
- Difficulty in walking
- Spastic paraplegia in the late stage
- Convulsion
- Death in extreme cases. It is due to rupture of aortic aneurysm caused by the toxin which affects the elasticity of the aorta, a condition called angiolathyrism.

ARGEMONE MEXICANA

The seeds of this plant are similar to mustard seeds. Mustard oil is often deliberately adulterated with seeds of argemone. Adulteration of mustard oil with oil of argemone causes a condition called epidemic dropsy and glaucoma. Argemone seeds are dark brown, globular with minute depressions and projections on the surface.
Active principle—Sanguinarine

Signs and symptoms
- Edema legs and generalized anasarca
- Dyspnea on slight exertion
- Hepatomegaly
- Hyperesthesia and tingling of limbs
- Knee jerk diminished or absent.

Cause of death: Heart failure. The toxin causes degenerative changes in cardiac muscles.

Postmortem findings
- Generalized anasarca
- Pedal edema
- Pleural effusion
- Pericardial effusion
- Enlarged liver
- Myocardial degeneration

Poisonous fish: The condition is called ichthyotoxicosis. It is due to presence of certain neurotoxins in the fish. Poisoning may also result from bacterial growth on decomposed fish. Example:
1. Great barracuda
2. Tunna
3. Red snapper
4. Shellfish
5. Calm

Signs and symptoms
- Nausea, vomiting and abdominal pain
- Burning in the throat
- Dilatation of pupil
- Hypotension
- Dyspnea
- Ascending motor and sensory paralysis

Cause of death—respiratory failure.

Postmortem findings—nonspecific.

Chemicals causing food poisoning
They are mainly food additives and pesticides.

   Food additives are: Coloring agent, flavoring agent, preservatives. Monosodium glutamate (MSG) is a flavoring agent. Though not confirmed, excessive intake may cause numbness of the limbs and trunk, bronchospasm, convulsion in children. They are not known to cause death.

Pharmaceutical Products

ANALGESICS

Acetylsalicylic Acid (Aspirin)

It is a white, odorless crystalline powder, commonly used as an analgesic and antipyretic.

Signs and symptoms
- Burning pain in throat and stomach
- Nausea, vomiting, sometimes diarrhea
- Vertigo, ringing in ears (tinnitus)
- Sweating and hyperthermia
- Vision impairment
- Dilated pupils
- Delirium and hallucination
- Proteinuria due to renal tubular necrosis
- Respiratory alkalosis

Cause of death
1. Respiratory failure
2. Uremia leading to circulatory failure.

Fatal dose: 15–20 gm. Blood level of 50 mg% is toxic and 100 mg% is fatal

Fatal period: A few minutes to a few hours.

Postmortem findings
- Rashes over skin
- Lungs are congested and edematous
- Subpleural hemorrhage
- Gastric mucosa show congestion
- Liver shows hepatitis
- Kidneys show evidence of acute tubular necrosis

Paracetamol (Acetaminophen)

It is the active metabolite of acetanilide and phenacetin. It is used as an antipyretic and has no anti-inflammatory properties. This poisoning is common in children.

Signs and symptoms
- Nausea, vomiting, abdominal pain.

- Tender liver with signs and symptoms of hepatotoxicity because of centrilobular necrosis of liver
- Renal tubular necrosis

Cause of death—hepatic failure

Fatal dose—10–20 gm

Fatal period—2–4 days

Postmortem findings
- Liver is enlarged
- Centrilobular necrosis of liver on histopathology
- Acute renal tubular necrosis on histopathology
- Necrotic changes in myocardium
- Cerebral edema

NSAIDS (NON-STEROIDAL ANTI-INFLAMMATORY DRUGS)

Examples of some of the common NSAIDs of various groups are:
Phenylbutazone, ibuprofen, ketoprofen, naproxen, mefenamic acid, indomethacin, ketorolac, diclofenac, aceclofenac, piroxicam and nimesulide

Signs and symptoms
The adverse effects of overdose of these drugs depending upon the types are
- Epigastric burning and pain
- Gastritis and abdominal pain
- Vomiting and diarrhea
- Vertigo and seizures
- Hypotension and bradycardia
- Respiratory distress and pulmonary edema
- Metabolic acidosis

Cause of death: Death is very rare.

Fatal dose: Mostly non-fatal. Only adverse effects as described above.

ANTIHISTAMINICS

Examples are diphenhydramine, promethazine, pheniramine, prochlorperazine meclizine, chlorpheniramine, triprolidine, cyclizine, terfenadine, astemizole cetirizine, loratidine, cinnarizine

Signs and symptoms
Adverse effects of over dosage because of CNS depression and anticholinergic properties are:
- Dryness of skin and mouth
- Somnolence (drowsiness)
- Blurred vision

- Vomiting, diarrhea or constipation depending on the drug
- Extrapyramidal (neuromuscular) disorder of dystonic or parkinsonic type. Commonly seen with prochlorperazine (stemetil)
- Cardiac arrhythmia are known to be caused by astemizole and terfenadine.

Cause of death: Non-fatal, only adverse effects

ANTIBIOTICS

There are various types of antibiotics. With the emergence of drug resistant bacteria, more and more newer antibiotics are added in the list.

Common groups are:
- Penicillins, e.g. ampicillin, amoxicillin, methicillin, piperacillin
- Aminoglycosides, e.g. amikacin, gentamycin, tobramycin, kanamycin
- Cephalosporins, e.g. cephalexin (1G), e.g. cephalexine, cefuroxime (2G), cefixime, cefotaxime, cefpodoxime cefpodoxime, ceftriaxone (3G), cefepime, cefluprenum (4G)
- Fluoroquinolones, e.g. ciprofloxacin, levofloxacin and ofloxacin
- Macrolide, e.g. erythromycin, azithromycin, roxithromycin, clarithromycin
- Tetracyclines, e.g. tetracycline, doxycycline, minocycline

Signs and symptoms
Adverse reaction varies from hypersensitivity, diarrhea, nephritis
- Skin rashes (with oral penicillins), anaphylaxis (with injectable penicillins)
- Cholestatic hepatitis (with erythromycin)
- Tinnitus, deafness, vertigo (with aminoglycosides)
- Vomiting, diarrhea, abdominal pain, coagulopathy (with cephalosporines),
- Abdominal pain, vomiting, diarrhea, yellowish discoloration of teeth of a child in the teething age group (with tetracycline)
- Nausea, vomiting, abdominal pain, headache, tendonitis, insomnia (with fluoroquinolones)

Cause of death
Except for anaphylactic reaction to injectable penicillin none of the oral antibiotics are fatal, but have adverse reactions in overdosage and sometimes even in therapeutic doses.

ANTIAMOEBIC DRUGS

Metronidazole

Signs and symptoms
In chronic poisoning
- Nausea, vomiting
- Metallic taste in mouth as it is secreted in saliva
- Vertigo
- Paraesthesia of hands and feet.
- Death due to metronidazole poisoning is unknown.

Anti-tubercular Drugs

INH (isonicotinic acid hydrazide)

Signs and symptoms of adverse effects
- Nausea, vomiting, stomachache
- Tingling and numbness in extremities due to peripheral neuropathy
- Hepatitis with associated symptoms
- Fever and rash

Ethambutol

Signs and symptoms of adverse effects
- Optic neuritis causing decreased visual acquity.
- Hyperuricemia causing arthralgia
- Hepatitis with associated symptoms
- Hepatic failure sometimes with fatal outcome which is the cause of death.

Rifampicin

Signs and symptoms of adverse effects
- Orange-red color urine, skin, mucus membrane, sweat and tears.
- Epigastric pain
- Diarrhea
- Headache
- Dizziness

Pyrazinamide
- Nausea, vomiting and anorexia
- Thrombocytopenia
- Sideroblastic anemia
- Erythroid hyperplasia
- Allergic manifestation as rash, itching, hives and swelling of lips

INSULIN POISONING

Insulin toxicity can be fatal. It can be suicidal, homicidal and rarely accidental. Insulin has no effect on body when taken orally.

Signs and symptoms of insulin overdose
- Cold and clammy skin with sweats
- Giddiness with confusion
- Tachycardia
- Visual disturbance
- Unconsciousness
- Death

Normal blood insulin level
Fasting—<25 ml IU/L, PP (2 hours after glucose intake) 16–166 ml IU/L

Fatal dose—Variable. A dose more than 200–300 units are fatal.

Postmortem findings

No specific findings.

- Needle marks, if any, should be preserved in a refrigerator or frozen.
- A control sample should be taken for comparison
- Presence of insulin and protamine (heparin antagonist) at the site of injection is significant.
- Frozen serum separated from RBCs should be sent for quantitative and qualitative analysis.
- Severe astrocyte proliferation with GFAP (glial fibrillary acid protein), IHC (immune histochemistry) is found in brain in insulin overdosage.
- Very low level of glucose is found in vitreous humor
- Insulin can also be recovered from bile by radioimmunoassay.

Household Poisons

Definition

There are various products present in a household that can lead to poisoning if not handled carefully.

Causes of Household Poisoning

• Accidental—usually seen in children below 5 years and careless adults.
• Storing some products close to food.
• Containers having some harmful substance with open lid.

Classification

Depending upon the place in a house
1. *Stores/attics*
   • Napthalline (moth) balls, insecticides, pesticides, rat poison, kerosene oil
2. *Kitchen*
   • Drain cleaners (NaOH, sulfuric acid)
   • Dish cleaners (sodium carbonate or washing soda, detergents)
3. *Bathroom*
   • Soap (sodium laureth sulfate, sodium palmitate, sodium olivate)
   • Shampoo (sodium lauryl sulfate which is a surfactant, dimethicone, citric acid, pantethol, cocamidopropyl betaine)
   • Hair oil—ingredients depend on the brand of oil (some contain glycerine stearate, isopropyl alcohol, panthenol, propylene glycol, etc. aloe vera plant extract, carnitine, olive oil, natural oils like coconut, amla, mustard, etc.)
4. *Bedroom*
   • Cosmetics (castor oil, tarrtazine, erythrocine, mineral mica, titanium dioxide, etc.)
   • Perfume (a mixture of aroma compounds, fixative, solvent)
   • Deodorants (aluminium compounds, paraben, propylene glycol, triclosan, etc.)
5. *Basement*
   • Paint thinner (acetone, turpentine, naptha, toluene, mineral spirit, etc.)
   • Paint remover (dichloromethane or DMC, calcium hydroxide, limonene)
   • Anti-freezes or coolant used in internal combustion engines (water and ethylene glycol)

Poisoning by petroleum products, pharmaceutical products and food poisoning are together classified under **domestic poisons.**

Petroleum Products

They are divided into two types
1. Hydrocarbons
2. Non-hydrocarbons
   Hydrocarbons are organic compounds that contain only carbon and hydrogen.

They are classified as:
1. Aliphatic
2. Aromatic

Examples of aliphatic hydrocarbon
a. Gaseous—methane, propane, butane
b. Liquid—kerosene, diesel, petrol

Signs and symptoms
- Characteristic odor specific to the hydrocarbon in the breath and vomitus.
- Pain and burning in throat
- Nausea, vomiting and abdominal pain
- Pupils constricted initially, become dilated later on
- Bronchopneumonia
- Cough, choking, dyspnea due to aspiration
- Hemoptysis in severe cases
- Sings of pulmonary edema
- Pink froth around mouth and nosrtils
- Drowsiness leading to coma

Cause of death: Respiratory failure.

Fatal dose: Depends on the substance.
Kerosene—10–15 ml.

Fatal period: Few hours–24 hours.

Postmortem findings
- Froth (sometimes blood tinged) around mouth and nostrils
- Characteristic odor of the type of hydrocarbon ingested
- Lungs edematous, increased weight. On cut section of the lungs there is oozing of bloody froth and bronchopneumonia
- Petechial hemorrhages on surface of lungs and heart.
- Stomach wall congested with hemorrhagic patches
- All the organs are highly congested

Signs and symptoms of household poisons

Compound	Type	Signs and symptoms
1. Dishwashing powder	Irritant	Irritation in mouth throat and stomach
2. Dishwashing liquid	Irritant	Retching, choking and violent cough
3. Detergents	Soaps	Vomiting
4. Hair dyes, shampoo, bath oil, hair conditioner	Non-toxic	May have vomiting

MCI Guidelines for Training in Forensic Medicine

The objective at the end of undergraduate training course in forensic medicine is that the student should:

1. Identify the basic medicolegal aspects of hospital and general practice.
2. Define the medicolegal responsibilities of a general physician while rendering community service either in a rural primary health centre or an urban health centre.
3. Appreciate the physician's responsibilities in criminal matters and respect for the codes of medical ethics.
4. Diagnose, manage and also identify legal aspects of common acute and chronic poisonings.
5. Describe the medicolegal aspects and findings of postmortem examination in case of death due to common unnatural conditions and poisonings.
6. Detect occupational and environmental poisoning, prevention and epidemiology of common poisoning and their legal aspects particularly pertaining to Workmen's Compensation Act.
7. Describe the general principles of analytical toxicology.
8. Medical jurisprudence in view of the Consumer Protection Act—wherein doctors have been covered under its ambit. They have both rights as well as responsibilities. Under Medical Insurance Acts of negligence covered as well as rights for effective service delivery. The MCI, however, has not specified the syllabus for theory and practical for undergraduate teaching curriculum in Forensic Medicine.

MCI GUIDELINES FOR COMPETENCY BASED POSTGRADUATE TRAINING PROGRAM FOR MD IN FORENSIC MEDICINE

The teaching and learning program has been defined. During the course of three years the students are assessed every year on the basis of their performance. The combined assessment at the end of three years is taken as their internal assessment. The following are the teaching and learning methods for postgraduate students of forensic medicine.

Teaching Methodology

1. *Lectures:* Lectures are to be kept to a minimum. They may, however, be employed for teaching certain topics. Lectures may be didactic or integrated. The course shall be of three years, organized in six units (0–5). This modular pattern is a guideline for the department, to organize training. Training program can be modified depending upon the work load and academic assignments of the department.

2. *Journal Club and subject seminars:* Both are recommended to be held once a week. All the PG students are expected to attend and actively participate in discussion and enter in the Log Book relevant details. Further, every PG trainee must make a presentation from the allotted journal(s), selected articles and a total of 12 seminar presentations in three years. The presentations would be evaluated and would carry weightage for internal assessment.
3. *Case presentations:* Minimum of 5 cases to be presented by every PG trainee each year. They should be assessed using checklists and entries made in the log book.
4. Clinico-pathological correlation/conference: Recommended once a month for all postgraduate students. Presentation is to be done by rotation. If cases are not available, it could be supplemented by published CPCs.
5. *Inter-departmental meetings:* These meetings should be attended by postgraduate students and relevant entries must be made in the Log Book.
6. *Teaching skills:* The postgraduate students shall be required to participate in the teaching and training programme of undergraduate students and interns.
7. Undertake audit, use information technology tools and carry out research, both basic and clinical, with the aim of publishing his work and presenting his work at various scientific fora.
8. *Continuing Medical Education (CME) Programmes:* At least two CME programmes should be attended by each student in 3 years.
9. *Conferences:* The student to attend courses, conferences and seminars relevant to the speciality.
10. A postgraduate student of a postgraduate degree course in broad specialities/superspecialities would be required to present one poster presentation, to read one paper at a national/state conference and to present one research paper which should be published/accepted for publication/sent for publication during the period of his postgraduate studies so as to make him eligible to appear at the postgraduate degree examination.
11. *Rotation:* Other than the Department of Forensic Medicine, student may be posted for training in the following clinical disciplines for a given period of time on rotational basis: Place of posting for first year, second year, third year respectively.
    1. Trauma and emergency/casualty/emergency medicine department—1 month, 15 days, 15 days
    2. Radiology—7 days, 5 days, 3 days
    3. Psychiatry—5 days, 3 days, 2 days
    4. Forensic science lab—7 days, 15 days, not required in 3rd year
    5. Histopathology—7 days, 5 days, 3 days

ASSESSMENT

Formative assessment during the training.

General principles: Internal assessment should be frequent, cover all domains of learning and use to provide feedback to improve learning; it should also cover professionalism and communication skills.

The internal assessment should be conducted in theory and clinical examination. Quarterly assessment during the MD training should be based on the following educational activities:

1. Journal based/recent advances learning
2. Patient based/laboratory or skill based learning
3. Self-directed learning and teaching
4. Departmental and interdepartmental learning activity
5. External and outreach activities/CMEs

The student to be assessed periodically as per categories listed in postgraduate student appraisal form as set in the guidelines.

SUMMATIVE ASSESSMENT

The summative examination would be carried out as per the Rules given in Postgraduate Medical Education Regulations, 2000. The examination shall be in three parts:

1. Thesis

Thesis shall be submitted at least six months before the theory and clinical/practical examination. The thesis shall be examined by a minimum of three examiners—one internal and two external examiners, who shall not be the examiners for theory and practical examination. A PG trainee shall be allowed to appear for the theory and practical/clinical examination only after the acceptance of the thesis by the examiners.

2. Theory

The examinations shall be organized on the basis of 'Grading 'or 'Marking system' to evaluate and to certify PG trainee's level of knowledge, skill and competence at the end of the training. Obtaining a minimum of 50% marks in 'Theory' as well as 'Practical' separately shall be mandatory for passing examination as a whole. The examination for MD shall be held at the end of 3rd academic year. An academic term shall mean six month's training period. There shall be four papers each of three hours duration.

These are:

Theory examination: There shall be four theory papers.

Paper I: Basic of forensic medicine, basic sciences and allied subjects.

Paper II: Clinical forensic medicine and medical jurisprudence.

Paper III: Forensic pathology and toxicology.

Paper IV: Recent advances in forensic medicine, forensic psychiatry and medical toxicology, applied aspects of clinical disciplines and forensic sciences

3. Practical Examination

Practical examination would be spread over two days and should be as follows:

Day 1

- Clinical cases: (any 4) Age estimation, injury report, examination of an insane person to evaluate criminal/civil responsibility, examination of an intoxicated person, examination of a suspected case of poisoning (acute/chronic), disputed paternity case and sexual offences (accused and victim).
- Spots (10) Histopathology slides, photographs, exhibit material, X-rays, mounted specimens, bones, poisons and weapons, charts, etc.

- Toxicology exercises (02): Identification and details of common poisons or chemical tests, etc.
- Laboratory tests (01): Identification of biological stains (semen, blood, body fluids), histopathology slides of medicolegal relevance, gram and acid fast staining, etc.

Day 2

- Postmortem examination.
- Thesis/seminar presentation—for assessment of research/teaching ability
- Discussion on a case for expert opinion
- Grand viva voce.

Reader's Notes

Reader's Notes